W9-BXD-558

An Introduction
to Developmental
Disabilities

A Neurodevelopmental Perspective

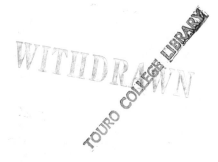
WITHDRAWN
TOURO COLLEGE LIBRARY

WS
368
B877
1994

$34.95

Singular 95-311

4/24/95

A9503749

AN INTRODUCTION TO DEVELOPMENTAL DISABILITIES

A NEURODEVELOPMENTAL PERSPECTIVE

WITHDRAWN

EDITED BY

FRANK R. BROWN, III, Ph.D., M.D.
Professor of Pediatrics
Baylor College of Medicine
Director, Meyer Center
for Developmental Pediatrics
Texas Children's Hospital
Houston, Texas

NICK ELKSNIN, Ph.D., NCSP
Adjunct Professor of Education
The Citadel
Charleston, South Carolina

SINGULAR PUBLISHING GROUP, INC.
SAN DIEGO, CALIFORNIA

Singular Publishing Group, Inc.
4284 41st Street
San Diego, California 92105-1197

© 1994 by Singular Publishing Group, Inc.

Typeset in 10/12 Times by ExecuStaff
Printed in the United States of America by McNaughton & Gunn

All rights, including that of translation, reserved. No part of this
publication may be reproduced, stored in a retrieval system, or
transmitted in any form or by any means, electronic, mechanical,
recording, or otherwise, without the prior written permission of
the publisher.

Library of Congress Cataloging-in-Publication Data

Brown, Frank R., III, 1943–
     An introduction to developmental disabilities : a
neurodevelopmental perspective / by Frank R. Brown, III, Nick
Elksnin.
          p.   cm.
     Includes bibliographical references and index.
     ISBN 1-56593-103-3
     1. Developmentally disabled children.   I. Elksnin, Nick.
II. Title
RJ506.D47B76   1994
618.92—dc20   94-7358
                                                       CIP

CONTENTS

Preface   ix

Contributors   xi

CHAPTER 1 **The Child With Developmental
           Disabilities: Developing a Generalist's
           Perspective**   1

The Physician as Generalist   2
Neurodevelopmental History   3
Neurodevelopmental Examination   10
Factors To Be Considered When Interpreting
    Neurodevelopment   20
Developmental Disabilities/Neurodevelopmental
    Principles   21
Conclusion   28

CHAPTER 2 **Children With Motor Impairment**   29

Patterns of Normal Motor Function   30
Patterns of Motor Dysfunction/Tonal Difficulties   46

Patterns of Motor Dysfunction/Dyscoordination
and Extraneous Movements   **52**
Motor Assessment   **55**
Intervention   **56**
Conclusion   **57**

CHAPTER 3   **Children With Cognitive Impairment**   **59**
Components of Cognition   **60**
Factors Affecting Cognitive Function   **67**
Cognitively Based Disorders   **68**
Assessment Strategies and Clinical Issues   **81**
Conclusion   **83**

CHAPTER 4   **Children With Speech, Language,
and Hearing Impairment**   **85**
Terminology   **86**
Identification   **86**
Hearing   **87**
Overview of Speech Systems   **101**
Language   **107**
Conclusion   **119**

CHAPTER 5   **Children With Developmental
Disabilities: Analysis and
Modification of Behavior Problems**   **121**
The Basics of a Behavior Analytic Approach
to Behavior Problems   **124**
Applications to Typical Behavior Problems   **127**
Functional Analysis   **133**
Response Classes   **137**
Children With Autism and Pervasive
Developmental Disorder   **141**
Extensions   **146**
Conclusion   **150**

CHAPTER 6   **Children With Developmental
Disabilities: Family Issues**   **153**
Family Characteristics   **154**

Family Interaction   **156**
Family Functions   **159**
Family Life Cycle   **161**
Stages of Parental Reaction to Diagnosis
   of Disability   **163**
Other Aspects of Parental Reaction   **165**
Explaining the Diagnosis to Parents   **166**

CHAPTER 7   **The Spectrum of Developmental
            Disabilities**   **169**
Case 1   **170**
Case 2   **176**

Glossary   **187**

References   **193**

Index   **213**

PREFACE

Developmental disabilities, defined as chronic, neurologically based limiting conditions, occur rather commonly. Mental retardation and cerebral palsy, for example, affect approximately 3% and 0.2% of children nationally, respectively. Learning disabilities, as more subtle developmental problems, affect even larger numbers of children, variously estimated as 10–15% of children. Based simply on frequency of occurrence then, it is important that physicians and allied health professionals working with children be well versed in identification and treatment of these and related chronic disabling disorders.

Many parents and professionals envisage children with developmental disabilities as severely impaired in single aspects of cognitive or motor function. In fact, most children with developmental disabilities have subtle dysfunction in multiple developmental domains. This can be best understood through recognition that developmental disabilities stem from brain damage and that central nervous system insults in children are diffuse in distribution and mild in extent. The "typical" child with a developmental disability should then be anticipated, until proven otherwise, to have dysfunction in multiple developmental domains.

In addition to neurologically based deficits, children with developmental disabilities frequently have associated behavioral and emotional problems. Professionals attending children with developmental disabilities need to consider the total child and interactions among these problem areas. The authors believe that an interdisciplinary approach provides the most thorough understanding of a child with multiple areas of dysfunction. We therefore address topics in an interdisciplinary format hoping to convey how dysfunction in one developmental domain can interact with dysfunction in other domains to produce the various profiles observed in children with developmental disabilities. At the same time, we encourage understanding of some basic neurodevelopmental principles that we believe transcend discipline-specific approaches and facilitate adoption of what we term a "generalist's perspective." We hope this combination of an interdisciplinary and generalist's approach will help the reader develop a broad-based and integrated perspective on the variety of dysfunctions that can arise in children with developmental disabilities.

Finally, we hope this text will serve as an introduction and provide a background for understanding more detailed treatises on individual aspects of these children.

CONTRIBUTORS

Kimberlee Berry-Sawyer, Ph.D.
Department of Psychiatry and
   The Clinical Center for the
   Study of Development and
   Learning
University of North Carolina
   School of Medicine
Chapel Hill, North Carolina

Michael F. Cataldo, Ph.D.
Professor
Department of Psychiatry and
   Behavioral Sciences
The Johns Hopkins University
   School of Medicine
Kennedy Krieger Institute
Baltimore, Maryland

Linda K. Elksnin, Ph.D.
Professor
Coordinator of Graduate Special
   Education Programs

The Citadel
Charleston, South Carolina

Stephen R. Hooper, Ph.D.
Associate Professor
Department of Psychiatry and
   The Clinical Center for the
   Study of Development and
   Learning
University of North Carolina
   School of Medicine
Chapel Hill, North Carolina

Janice Howard, Ph.D.
Department of Psychiatry and
   The Clinical Center for the
   Study of Development and
   Learning
University of North Carolina
   School of Medicine
Chapel Hill, North Carolina

George W. Hynd, Ph.D.
Professor of Educational
  Psychology and Psychology
University of Georgia
Athens, Georgia

Rebecca Landa, Ph.D., CCC-SLP
Assistant Professor of Psychiatry
Director, Communication
  Disorders Clinic
Co-Director, Autism Research
  Program
The Johns Hopkins University
  School of Medicine
Baltimore, Maryland

Frederick List, Ph.D.
Department of Psychiatry and
  The Clinical Center for the
  Study of Development and
  Learning
University of North Carolina
  School of Medicine
Chapel Hill, North Carolina

James Miedaner, M.S., PT
Associate Director of Physical
  Therapy
University of Wisconsin Hospital
  and Clinics
Madison, Wisconsin

Jean A. Patz, M.S., OTR
Department of Occupational
  Therapy and Private Practice
  in Pediatrics
Towson State University
Baltimore, Maryland

Keith J. Slifer, Ph.D.
Assistant Professor
Department of Psychiatry and
  Behavioral Sciences
The Johns Hopkins University
  School of Medicine
Kennedy Krieger Institute
Baltimore, Maryland

Jane A. Summers, Ph.D.
Assistant Professor
Department of Psychiatry and
  Behavioral Sciences
The Johns Hopkins University
  School of Medicine
Kennedy Krieger Institute
Baltimore, Maryland

Robert G. Voigt, M.D.
Assistant Professor of Pediatrics
Baylor College of Medicine/
  Texas Children's Hospital
Houston, Texas

**Michael K. Wynne, Ph.D.,
  CCC-A/SLP**
Associate Professor
Department of Otolaryngology
Indiana University School of
  Medicine
Indianapolis, Indiana

ACKNOWLEDGMENT

To our wives, Mitten and Linda, and to Reggie and Riggs Brown.

C H A P T E R   1

THE CHILD WITH DEVELOPMENTAL DISABILITIES: DEVELOPING A GENERALIST'S PERSPECTIVE

Frank R. Brown, III, Ph.D., M.D.

The authors of this text share several basic neurodevelopmental principles in our approach to children with developmental disabilities. In the present chapter we introduce these principles, and we will return to them in subsequent chapters as we discuss the spectrum of developmental disorders. It is our hope that an understanding and acceptance of these neurodevelopmental principles will help readers subvert their discipline-specific approaches to what we term a "generalist's perspective." This broader, less discipline-specific, approach should enhance individual professionals' understanding of developmental disabilities and provide a framework for an interdisciplinary approach to assessment and prescriptive plan development and application.

A second topic introduced in this chapter is the generalist's approach to elicitation of a temporal history of development (neurodevelopmental history) and performance of a neurodevelopmental examination.

The approach discussed is truly a generalist's approach in the sense that perspectives on development obtained through the neurodevelopmental history and examination can serve as a basis for more detailed examinations by professionals in the fields of developmental medicine, psychology, speech-language pathology, and physical and occupational therapy.

THE PHYSICIAN AS GENERALIST

There are several factors that lead us to suggest that the physician is ideally positioned to function as a generalist in the identification and management of children with developmental disabilities. First is the simple fact that the physician is typically the initial professional resource contacted by families with questions regarding their child's developmental progress. Second is that the physician, by virtue of early and ongoing contact with families, has knowledge of pre- and perinatal factors that potentially place a child at increased risk for subsequent developmental problems. A final consideration relates to the fact that children with developmental disabilities have diffuse neurological, behavioral, and emotional problems and are frequently best served by an interdisciplinary team of health care professionals. The physician, with broad-based training in neurological, behavioral, and emotional aspects of children and families, is well suited to integrate team findings and recommendations and can present them in a balanced, intelligible perspective to a family.

The combination of these factors leads us to the conclusion that the physician is ideally positioned to function as a generalist in the early identification and management of children with developmental disabilities. This does not preclude a generalist's perspective being adopted by other disciplines. In fact, we believe colleagues can enhance their contributions to the interdisciplinary process through incorporation of generalist perspectives, including adoption of the neurodevelopmental history and examination format to be described. It should be understood, then, in the discussion to follow that in many circumstances the terms "physician" and "generalist" can appropriately be interchanged.

To make these contributions to the early diagnostic and interdisciplinary management process, the physician must expand the traditional role of medical history taking and physical examination to include a neurodevelopmental history and neurodevelopmental examination. The neurodevelopmental history is the temporal accounting of a child's development to date across four major developmental domains (Gesell & Amatruda, 1947), including:

1. Motor—including gross, fine, and oral motor function.
2. Visual perceptual/problem solving—including concepts such as size, shape, and spatial relationships.
3. Language—including expressive and receptive language abilities.
4. Social-adaptive—including self-help skills such as dressing and feeding.

The *neurodevelopmental examination* is the examination of a child's quantitative and qualitative development in these same domains. The physician embarks in examination of a child through the neurodevelopmental history and examination, although some of the same areas will be reviewed by colleagues in developmental and behavioral psychology, physical and occupational therapy, and speech-language pathology. The physician does this, not because other professionals are not "trusted," but rather to ensure the physician's generalist perspective in the interdisciplinary diagnostic and therapeutic evaluative process. Components of the neurodevelopmental history and neurodevelopmental examination are addressed next.

NEURODEVELOPMENTAL HISTORY

Utility of the Neurodevelopmental History

The neurodevelopmental history, as a temporal accounting of development to date in motor, visual perception/problem solving, language, and social-adaptive domains, is an important part of the generalist's approach to children with developmental disabilities and has many important utilities. Chief among these is the discrimination the history affords the generalist in establishing "patterns" of developmental delay and especially if there is any element of progression of the disability. A developmental history reflecting a constant, albeit slower than normal rate of developmental progress, will be consistent with a "static encephalopathy"; whereas a history suggesting a slowing in the rate of developmental progress over time will be consistent with a "progressive" or "neurodegenerative encephalopathy." Though progressive neurological disorders are rare as causes of developmental delays (approximately 2–3% of severe and profound developmental delays), the conditions assume increased importance, because:

a. The family can sometimes be given a precise causation for the child's problems.

   b. Many progressive neurological disorders are genetically inherited
   and recurrence can be prevented through genetic counseling.
   c. Specific therapies are available for some progressive neurological disorders.

The astute generalist can utilize a neurodevelopmental history to identify progressive neurological disorders at the earliest possible age and
can, thereby, help prevent recurrence and promote early institution of
appropriate therapies.

The physician can utilize the neurodevelopmental history to assist
in deciding what, if any, additional diagnostic tests are needed. A
history suggesting a constant, although slower than normal rate of developmental progress ("static encephalopathy"), may disincline the physician from performing elaborate studies to establish causation. The
yield of such efforts, both from the standpoint of establishing causation and of identifying treatable disorders, is usually limited. On the
other hand, a history consistent with a falloff in the rate of neurodevelopment ("progressive" or "neurodegenerative encephalopathy") should
alert the physician to perform a variety of additional diagnostic tests
(e.g., computed tomography, nuclear magnetic resonance scans, electro-
encephalogram, urine metabolic screen, serum/urinary amino acids,
biochemical evaluations of cultured skin fibroblasts, and the like). By
restricting use of such diagnostic studies to potentially progressive or
neurodegenerative processes as identified in the neurodevelopmental
history, the physician can optimally identify those children whose course
is expected to be altered by use of this information.

The neurodevelopmental history affords the generalist a temporal
accounting of developmental progress to date, and serves as a guide-
line to appropriate levels at which to begin the neurodevelopmental examination (cf. following). Consistency observed between the history and
examination yields increasing reliability and validity in conclusions regarding levels of neurodevelopmental function.

Finally, the neurodevelopmental history allows the generalist to
compare the parents' accounting of developmental history with developmental findings during the neurodevelopmental examination, to gain
insight into how realistic the parents are in their understanding of the
extent of their child's problems. This information can help guide subsequent parent conferences and counseling sessions.

Prenatal and Perinatal Risk Factors

Through a carefully elicited pregnancy, labor, and birth history, the physician can identify pre- and perinatal risk factors that potentially place

a child at-risk for subsequent developmental disabilities. Some of these risk factors are outlined in Table 1–1.

In equating high-risk situations with subsequent developmental disabilities, the physician must appreciate that many children with developmental disabilities may not have a readily identifiable history of such difficulties. In fact, although many children with a high-risk pre- and/or perinatal course will manifest with subsequent neurological deficits, the majority of children with neurological deficits do not have histories that would be identified as high-risk. This reflects that many of the "risk factors" listed in Table 1–1 manifest in subtle, sometimes

TABLE 1–1. Prenatal and perinatal history—risk factors associated with developmental disabilities.

Pregnancy	Labor and Delivery (cont'd)
Maternal age	Problems:
Paternal age	premature rupture of membranes
Parity	maternal fever
Length of gestation	toxemia
Maternal weight gain	abnormal bleeding
Fetal activity	fetal monitoring
Previous maternal obstetrical	failure of labor to progress
problems	labor induced
Problems:	Caesarian section
bleeding/spotting	forceps/instrumentation
medications	resuscitation
trauma	abnormalities at birth
toxemia	abnormal placenta
radiation	
rash/infection	**Neonatal**
fluid retention	Duration of hospitalization
abnormal fetal movements	Problems:
alcohol	respiratory distress syndrome
tobacco	cyanosis
	seizures
Labor and Delivery	oxygen therapy
Hospital	feeding problems
Duration of labor	infections
Birth weight	jaundice
Apgars	metabolic
Analgesia/sedation	congenital abnormalities
Presentation	apnea

undetectable fashion, and there are presumably a number of risk fac-tors of which we are currently unaware and that ultimately will belong on any such list.

In essence, we are inferring that our current technologies are not sophisticated enough to pick up the potential impact of these more subtle insults. For example, although the effects of high maternal alco-hol consumption on the fetus and the full-blown fetal alcohol syndrome are obvious (intrauterine and postnatal growth retardation, physical abnormalities, and impaired cognitive development), the effects on the developing fetus of lesser degrees of alcohol and cigarette consump-tion, as well as other factors like subclinical maternal viral infections are far less known now. The presence of risk factors in a pregnancy, labor, and delivery should put the physician on early alert that subse-quent neurological development should be carefully monitored, and we hope that in the future the ability to identify milder (and more fre-quently occurring) insults will improve.

Parents as Historians

Besides the history questions used to identify high-risk pregnancies, the physician should elicit a careful history of temporal patterns of neuro-development across the four major domains of development outlined above, specifically: motor, visual perception/problem solving, language, and social-adaptive function. Although it might seem that the neuro-developmental history would evolve rather directly from the parental recounting of the course of development in each of these domains, many factors complicate this process.

The generalist needs to appreciate that parents will generally give the best neurodevelopmental history if they are asked to recount what they perceive as major events in their child's life (e.g., the age at which the child took first steps), and if they are asked to relate events that are more temporally current. It is important that questions be asked in the proper sequence to build the parents' confidence in their ability to relate historic details. The generalist can then expand the history to potentially more important areas such as receptive language and visual perception/problem solving. In these more important, but difficult ar-eas for the parents, it is important to ask questions from several dif-ferent perspectives and to be a bit persistent in the process.

Because some developmental domains are closely interrelated and overlap, the history-taking process is further complicated. Questions re-garding development of visual perception/problem solving are especially difficult for parents to recall, and questions in this domain need to be asked in a way that parents commonly observe and appreciate. This might translate into questions about development of skills related to everyday living, such as dressing and feeding. These "social-adaptive" skills, in turn, are dependent on fine motor development. Because of such complex interactions between different developmental domains, it becomes important for the generalist to dissociate data from the history into how much dysfunction stems from one developmental area as opposed to another.

The generalist needs to appreciate that when parents are asked to recount developmental milestones for a child with significant developmental delays, not only will development over time be protracted (quantitative variation), but also the quality of the process will be affected (qualitative variation). The combined protraction and blurring of evolution of skills contributes to parents' difficulties in readily recounting a neurodevelopmental history for their significantly delayed child.

Finally, parents are sensitive about their child's neurodevelopment being viewed as a rote compendium of deficits. The generalist should therefore develop the history via questions focused exclusively on age-equivalent descriptors, such as, "at what age did your child walk independently?" The generalist should avoid questions that imply perceptions of delay, such as, "when did you appreciate your child's delay in walking?" Terms that imply delayed development, such as "slow," "delayed," "retarded," "disabled," and "cerebral palsied" should be assiduously avoided because they promote miscommunication. These summary descriptors really serve no purpose at this time other than to potentially offend and distort the history-taking process. They are not nearly as useful as age-equivalent descriptors that enhance clearer communication between parent and physician.

Obtaining the Neurodevelopmental History

In practice, the neurodevelopmental history is best initiated by asking parents questions in the two areas of development in which they are anticipated to be the best observers—specifically gross motor development and expressive language (i.e., "walking" and "talking"). Some typical gross motor developmental milestones are summarized in Table 1–2. The generalist will next ask questions related to the temporal sequence of language and visual perceptual/fine motor development as outlined in Tables 1–3 and 1–4. As noted, a particularly difficult developmental domain for the parents to recount is visual perceptual/fine motor development. Parents might be asked to recount development of social-adaptive skills such as dressing and feeding and, to the extent

TABLE 1-2. Gross motor developmental milestones.

Age	Skill Attained
2 mo	Lifts head in face down (prone) posture
3 mo	Up on forearms in prone
4 mo	Up on wrists in prone
	Rolls over, face down (prone) to face up (supine)
5 mo	Rolls over, supine to prone
6 mo	Sits without support, anterior propping
8 mo	Lateral propping in sitting
	Lateralizes (reaches to side) in sitting
9 mo	Pulls to standing, cruises holding on
12 mo	Walks independently
	Posterior propping in sitting
18 mo	Runs
27 mo	Walks up stairs ("marking time")
3 yr	Pedals tricycle
	Walks up stairs alternating feet, down "marking time"
3.5 yr	Walks up and down stairs alternating feet
4.5 yr	Balances briefly (5 sec.) either foot
5 yr	Skips

such skills depend on perceptual and fine motor function, development in this domain can be inferred.

The generalist should conclude the history-taking process by asking the parents to state perceptions of their child's overall level of neurodevelopmental function in terms of age equivalents. This question can be as simple as "at what age level do you see your child functioning overall?" If the parents show resistance in formulating a response, the question could be restated "give me your best guess." If both parents are present, the question should be asked separately to determine concurrence (this concurrence may be of import later during parent conferencing). Further clarification is afforded if the parents are asked to describe age equivalents for areas of "best function" and "worst function." These efforts to encourage the parents to state their perceptions are a paradigm in eliminating a natural evolution of parental denial if the generalist opens a discussion with conclusions about developmental delays. If the generalist falls into the trap of placing conclusions about developmental delays on the table before the parents state

TABLE 1-3. Language—expressive and receptive milestones.

Age	Skill Attained
2 mo	Spontaneous smile
3 mo	Cooing (vowel) sounds
4 mo	Turns to voice
5 mo	Lateralizes to bell "Raspberry" or "Bronx Cheer"
6 mo	Babbling (consonant) sounds
7 mo	Orients to bell (2 planes)
8 mo	Ma-Ma/Da-Da, non-specific
9 mo	Gesture language (bye-bye, point to wants) Orients to bell (directly)
10 mo	Ma-Ma/Da-Da, specific
12 mo	First word other than ma-ma/da-da
14 mo	Follows 1-step command with gesture
16 mo	Follows 1-step command without gesture
18 mo	Indicates 1 body part 12 word vocabulary
21 mo	Combines 2 words 20 word vocabulary
24 mo	Follows 2-step command without gestures e.g., "Put the ball on the table and give the pencil to me" 50 word vocabulary
30 mo	Concept of "just one" Prepositions "on" & "under"
3 yr	Asks for word meanings Answers "What do you do when you're hungry?" Identifies sex Concepts of "big" & "little" Prepositions "behind" & "next to" 250 word vocabulary
4 yr	Tells stories using complex syntax Answers "What do you do when you're cold?" Concepts of "longer" & "shorter"
5 yr	Follows 3-step command in correct order Vocabulary too numerous to count

TABLE 1–4. Visual perceptual/fine motor milestones.

Age	Skill Attained
3 mo	Unfisted hands Active reaching
6 mo	Transfers hand-to-hand
8 mo	Holds 2 objects simultaneously
9 mo	Pincer grasp Finger feeds
12 mo	Drinks from cup Intentional release
14 mo	Spoon feeds
18 mo	Scribbles spontaneously
27 mo	Imitates horizontal/vertical stroke
3 yr	Unbuttons
4 yr	Buttons up
5 yr	Ties Shoes

their perceptions, denial will be a certainty. In other words, it's best that conclusions regarding developmental delays come out of the parent's (as opposed to the generalist's) "mouth."

Having obtained estimates of current neurodevelopmental functioning, for example, age equivalents through the neurodevelopmental history, the generalist will progress to the neurodevelopmental examination. Considering that neurodevelopment, even in the face of significant delays of development, is most typically of constant velocity, the generalist can extrapolate from the developmental history the current level of developmental function in each developmental domain. If the neurodevelopmental history has been carefully performed, the neurodevelopmental examination should simply confirm levels of neurodevelopmental function inferred in the history. The combination of the history and examination will produce a reliable and valid assessment.

NEURODEVELOPMENTAL EXAMINATION

Physicians have typically used "screening instruments" as a basis for identifying children with developmental disabilities and in making decisions regarding referrals for more detailed evaluations. Problems in using any unitary screening instrument include:

1. Results may produce significant false positives and negatives and referral decisions made solely on the basis of such screening are very apt to be inappropriate.
2. Instrumental design and use affords a limited perspective on neurodevelopment at only one point in time. This contrasts with and ignores the important utility of the developmental history and contributes to false positives and negatives.
3. Instrumental design affords no inherent reliability or validity of observation unless another instrument is employed to cross-check results.
4. Reliance on screening instruments translates into "test scores," with poor appreciation of the process used by the generalist in looking at neurodevelopment.

We feel that assessment and referral decisions are best made on the basis of appreciation of normal and abnormal development, the depth and breadth of training of the generalist, and the reliability and validity inherent in the neurodevelopmental history and examination gathering process. The neurodevelopmental examination described in this section is not intended to replace more detailed evaluations by allied health professionals; however, the combination of the neurodevelopmental examination and the neurodevelopmental history can help the generalist develop appropriate schema for subsequent referrals.

The neurodevelopmental examination is the physician's detailed examination of a child's development in at least three of the four areas discussed previously: motor (gross/fine/oral), visual perception and problem solving, and language (expressive/receptive). Social-adaptive function, for example, self-help skills such as dressing and feeding, is usually not directly assessed in the neurodevelopmental examination because of time constraints and lack of efficiency.

The physician performs the traditional physical examination in an orderly and rapport building sequence. This process assumes even more importance in the neurodevelopmental examination, with which we are purporting to examine cognitive and motor capacity. The success of this process frequently depends on deciding whether apparent disabilities represent true dysfunction or unwillingness to engage in the tasks ("can't do" vs. "won't do"). In attempting to resolve this critical issue, it is important that the examination be structured to optimize the child's performance. This, in turn, means that the child should be initially examined in areas of anticipated relative success and that the process be initiated at or below a level at which success is anticipated. By building rapport with the child, the examiner increases reliability and validity of the results.

Utilizing information from the neurodevelopmental history, the astute generalist will anticipate areas of possible significant dysfunction before initiating the examination. To optimize the child's performance in the neurodevelopmental examination, information gleaned in the history should be employed in selecting appropriate initial areas of assessment. Rapport is enhanced by careful selection of initial areas and levels of assessment to avoid challenging the child in areas of relative weakness early in the examination. Therefore, the generalist initiates the neurodevelopmental examination in areas of relative strength. For many children visual problem solving is an ideal starting point, because test items are high-interest tasks and are similar to children's play. Our experience suggests that it is usually best to initially avoid unnecessary levels of language demand, especially if the neurodevelopmental history suggests significant weaknesses in this area.

Assessment of Visual Perceptual/Problem Solving Abilities

In the neurodevelopmental examination, primary focus should be placed on those aspects of development that are most predictive of ultimate function. These are the cognitive areas of visual perception/problem solving and language understanding (receptive language). Assessment of visual perception/problem solving involves analysis of play-like skills with simple toy items such as the 1-inch cubes and pencil/crayons and paper described in Table 1–5. Because skills with these two items cover a broad range of developmental abilities (the cube activities cover a neurodevelopmental age range of 3 months to 7 years, and pencil/crayons and paper activities a range of 16 months to 12 years) and are so readily available, we advocate that the generalist, at a minimum, should survey a child's responses with these items.

When assessing a child's visual perceptual/problem solving abilities with 1-inch cubes, the examiner first builds the block construct out of the child's field of view (typically by covering the assembly process with the examiner's hand). The child is then given the appropriate number of blocks to build a duplicate of the examiner's model, and the model is left in place for visual imitation by the child. The two exceptions to this procedure are the staircase assemblies (Table 1–5[f] and [g]), in which the model is built out of the child's sight, shown to the child and then destroyed, with the child asked to build the assembly from visual memory.

The drawing tasks listed in Table 1–5 are suitable for testing visual perceptual development over a wide age range. The Gesell figures (Figure 1–1) are a series of increasingly complex figures that the child

TABLE 1–5. Assessment of visual perception/problem solving.

One-Inch Cubes (3 months to 7 years)

3 mo	Regards (visually tracks) cube
5 mo	Reaches up to obtain cube in supine (lying face up)
6 mo	Reaches out to obtain cube in sitting Transfers cube hand-to-hand
8 mo	Holds two cubes simultaneously
9 mo	Releases cube into a cup (over side of cup)
12 mo	Intentional (precise) release of cube into a cup
14 mo	Holds three cubes simultaneously
18 mo	Vertical tower of 3 cubes (a)
24 mo	Train of 3 cubes (b)
27 mo	Train of 4 cubes with smoke stack (c)
36 mo	3 block bridge (d)
4 yr	5 block gate (e)
5 yr	6 block staircase (f)
7 yr	10 block staircase (g)

Pencil and Paper (16 months to 12 years)

16 mo	Scribbles in imitation
18 mo	Scribbles spontaneously
27 mo	Imitates horizontal/vertical stroke
30 mo	Copies circle as circular motion
3 yr	Copies circle
3.5 yr	Copies cross
4 yr	Copies square
5 yr	Copies triangle
6 yr	Copies "Union Jack"
7 yr	Copies diamond
8 yr	Copies Maltese cross
9 yr	Copies cylinder
12 yr	Copies cube

Gesell Drawings
(see Figure 1–1)

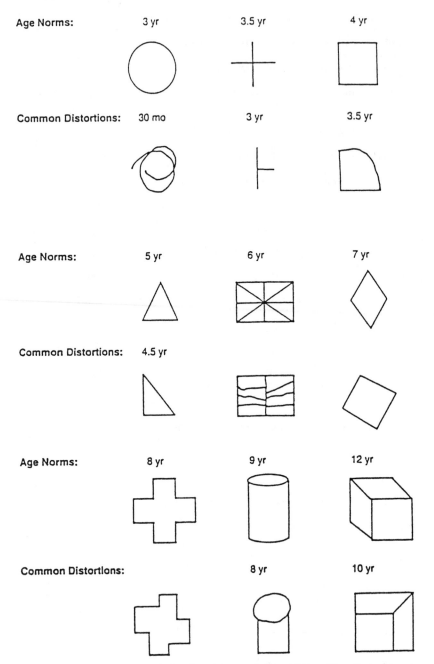

FIGURE 1-1. Assessment of visual-problem solving abilities (Gesell drawings).

is asked to replicate with crayon or pencil and paper. These drawings are presented to the child in a completed, predrawn fashion and the child is asked to draw a likeness of the figures. It is imperative that the generalist observe the child while replicating the figures, as satisfactory replication is not the only information to be gained. It is important to analyze the child's approach to replication of the figures, including areas like time required to complete the figures and omission of key elements. The child who does not understand the gestalt of the figures may, for example, approach a drawing like the "Union Jack" in a fragmented fashion, perhaps drawing it as a series of small triangles. Unless the child is observed in the drawing process, these qualitative deficits in performance may not be appreciated. Some of the most common distortions of the Gesell drawings are included in Figure 1–1.

Assessment of Language Functioning

We have previously said that the neurodevelopmental examination should commence with cognitive assessment and subsequently proceed to analysis of motor skills. Within the cognitive assessment, we recommend starting with visual perception/problem solving, then proceeding to language. A good reason for conducting the examination in this order is to guard against the child who may have disproportionate delay in language functioning relative to other cognitive abilities. This approach is particularly advised when the parents' neurodevelopmental history suggests that there are such problems in language. It is our experience that if children with any significant degree of language delay are initially approached with any significant language demand, that further cooperation in the examining process is impaired.

Assessment of language functioning does not depend on specific test items of the type described above for assessment of visual perception/problem solving abilities. In assessing language development, the generalist should be most concerned with what might be termed connected language understanding and usage, which is the ability to express utterances and understand and follow directions in daily life. This most meaningful aspect of a child's language development can be assessed simply and appropriately by examination of ability to manipulate familiar objects on command (i.e., following simple directions, with and without gestures, and of increasing complexity) and ability to answer simple comprehension questions listed in Table 1–3. Instruments such as the *Peabody Picture Vocabulary Test-Revised (PPVT-R)* (Dunn & Dunn, 1981) assess more limited aspects of language development (picture identification), and, therefore, may be less informative of meaningful language development. In other words, the generalist might well attach more meaning to the child's ability to comprehend the direction "put the book in the drawer" than the ability to identify pictures in the book, *PPVT-R*.

An important "red flag" in identifying language delay is the persistence of echolalia beyond approximately 30 months. Echolalia, as exemplified by the repetition of a question rather than responding to the question or echoing the last thing heard (e.g. Question—"Are you a boy or a girl?" Answer—"boy or girl" or "girl"), represents a failure to comprehend language. Its persistence beyond 30 months is tantamount to saying that the child is delayed in the language domain.

Within the context of an office setting it is unrealistic to expect a child to exhibit a reasonable facsimile of expressive vocabulary and mean length of utterance. To estimate expressive language, the generalist must rely in large part on the parents' history. This need not be a major deterrent to expressive language assessment if the examiner is aware that it is impossible for receptive language to lag expressive language development. On the other hand, expressive language, at least in the usual restricted evaluative setting, may well appear to lag receptive language development. Receptive language is, therefore, usually considered a far better indicator of inherent language capabilities. Finally, when encountering children with significant oral motor dysfunction that may affect oral language output, the generalist might use the developmental history of gesture language (e.g., pointing to communicate wants, waving bye-bye, and engaging in visual imitative games such as peek-a-boo) to gain insight into "expressive" language that is not dependent on oral motor function.

Assessment of Gross/Fine/Oral Motor Function

Having completed the cognitive (visual perceptual and language assessment) portion of the neurodevelopmental examination, the generalist will proceed with assessment of gross motor function. If the physician is the generalist, observation of gross motor function will be coupled with the traditional neurological examination, focusing on muscle mass, strength, tone, reflexes, coordination, and any soft neurological signs (mirror movements and synkinesis). These assessments are best reserved for the last part of the examination, because this is a more invasive aspect of the process—that is, the child is approached physically. By this point in the examination the child may very well be tired, and by reserving gross motor observation until after completion of assessment of cognitive function, cooperation will be optimized for the more critical cognitive areas. At the same time, the motor assessment may be perceived as fun, though the child might be tired.

The gross motor milestones listed in Table 1–2 can be used for guidelines in the neurodevelopmental examination of the motor areas. It is important to appreciate that some gross motor skills, for example ability to sit independently and to function in sitting, are attained over significant intervals of time. Reference to the sitting skills milestones listed in Table 1–2 reveals that sitting skills are attained over an approximate 6-month period, with ability to sit independently without support developing normally at approximately 6 months; whereas, more refined sitting skills (e.g., sitting with ability to catch oneself in a rearward fall with the arms) are only developed at approximately 12 months of age.

A child's ability to perform on stairs (see Table 1–2) can be a tool for assessing gross motor development, especially for children who are in an approximate 2.5- to 3.5-year level of gross motor function. At 2.5 years of gross motor development, a child can ascend stairs "marking time." At 3 years a child will ascend stairs by alternating feet, will descend stairs "marking time," and will have learned how to pedal. By 3.5 years a child will ascend and descend stairs with alternating feet.

As mentioned previously in the section on visual perceptual/fine motor assessment, an important antecedent to assessment of visual perceptual/problem solving abilities is determination of the extent of any intercurrent difficulties in fine motor performance. Assessment of these fine motor abilities is typically inferred from observation of a child's performance on visual problem solving tasks. An exact level of fine motor function is not derived from this process, rather an analysis of the extent to which fine motor difficulties might represent an interfering factor is inferred.

Oral motor functioning is inferred from the neurodevelopmental history and observation in such areas as feeding and speech articulation. Certainly a history of feeding difficulties and/or persistence of drooling suggests significant delays. An additional manifestation of oral motor dysfunction is delayed speech articulation. Children's speech should be nearly 100% intelligible to the parents by age 30 months and to strangers by 36 months.

Soft Neurological Signs

The classical neurological examination looks at what are termed _hard neurological signs_—that is, the neurological findings that are present or absent and are not modified by maturation of the child's nervous system. The presence or absence of such neurological findings is used to identify the presence of and allows localization of pathology in the nervous system. In the child's developing nervous system, the physician generalist examining a child is more typically presented with neurological findings that are on a developmental continuum—that is, they appear and disappear with development and maturation of the nervous system (Brown, Aylward, & Keogh, 1992). Pathology here does not equate simply with the presence or absence of physical findings, but depends on the extent of their presence and the timing of their appearance and disappearance. This has led to a great deal of confusion in interpreting the significance of these *soft neurological signs*. These soft neurological signs are most helpful in evaluating school-age children, with presence correlating significantly with learning disabilities.

Between one-third and one-half of children with learning problems (Brown et al., 1992) demonstrate significant soft neurological signs. Mirror movements and synkinesias (associated movements) represent the most commonly encountered soft neurological signs. Mirror movements are movements of an opposite extremity that arise when the examiner has made a specific request for isolated movement of one of the extremities. Synkinesias represent an overflow, or overshooting, of muscle movements into other surrounding muscle groups when the examiner has made a specific request for isolated movement of a particular muscle group. Both mirror movements and synkinesias are commonly encountered in children with learning disabilities, but their presence is not pathognomonic.

Short-term Memory Assessment

Short-term memory assessment is perhaps most relevant in evaluating school-age children having trouble following directions, in children experiencing difficulties with behavioral compliance, and in evaluation of children with possible attention-deficit hyperactivity disorder (ADHD). Assessment can be made through analysis of a child's ability to recall digits forward, digits reversed, and sentence memory (Table 1–6). Qualitative deviance may be noted if a child remembers the digits, but does not get them in the correct order (sequential memory deficit rather than a rote auditory memory deficit). Additionally, a child with ADHD frequently exhibits an inconsistent performance with digit recall, doing better when attention is focused carefully and distractions minimized. The child with ADHD also may exhibit better ability to reverse digits than to perform them forward.

TABLE 1-6. Auditory memory.

Digits Forward—Digits spaced approximately 1 second apart

2.5	yr	47	____	63	____	58	____
3	yr	641	____	352	____	837	____
4.5	yr	4729	____	3852	____	7261	____
7	yr	31589	____	48372	____	96183	____
10	yr	473859	____	429746	____	728394	____
Adult		72594836	____	47153962	____	41935826	____

Digits Reversed

7	yr	295	____	816	____	473	____
9	yr	8526	____	4937	____	3629	____
12	yr	81379	____	69582	____	52618	____
Adult		471952	____	583694	____	752618	____

Sentences—Read at a normal rate

4 yr   We are going to buy some candy for mother.
Jack likes to feed the little puppies in the barn.

5 yr   Jane wants to build a big castle in her playhouse.
Tom has lots of fun playing ball with his sister.

8 yr   Fred asked his father to take him to see the clowns in the circus.
Billy made a beautiful boat out of wood with his sharp knife.

11 yr   At the summer camp the children get up early in the morning and go swimming.
Yesterday we went for a ride in our car along the road that crosses the bridge.

13 yr   The airplane made a careful landing in the space which had been prepared for it.
Tom Brown's dog ran quickly down the road with a huge bone in his mouth.

Adult   The red headed woodpecker made a terrible fuss as they tried to drive the young away from the nest.
The early settlers had little idea of the great changes that were to take place in this country.

FACTORS TO BE CONSIDERED WHEN INTERPRETING NEURODEVELOPMENT

While using the neurodevelopmental history and examination to iden-tify children with developmental delays, the generalist should be aware of certain caveats:

1. Diagnoses of developmental delays should be based on com-binations of observations from the history and examination, rather than on a single assessment area.
2. There are normal familial patterns of developmental delays, such as late walkers within families of late walkers and late talkers within families of late talkers. Because some areas of development (language) are more important than others (gross motor), more attention should be paid to the late talker within the family of late talkers.
3. The generalist needs to be careful not to misconstrue "can't do" for "won't do." Obviously, if a child is tired or uncoop-erative, results of neurodevelopmental evaluation can be skewed. It is the generalist's responsibility to structure test items for maximum cooperation and engagement.
4. If the generalist discovers something that is at odds with the parents' accounting, it should be assumed, until proven other-wise, that something is discrepant in the testing. The parents may be poor observers or less than objective reporters, but this happens much less often than thought and should not be assumed.
5. With premature infants, physicians have traditionally compared developmental findings with "corrected" chronological age, in other words, within the first year of life, months of prematu-rity are subtracted from the chronological age for developmental comparisons. We recommend that this procedure be discarded in favor of simply talking about what the child is doing and that this not be related to any corrected age. The danger in comparing findings with corrected ages is that significant de-grees of developmental delay may be incorrectly minimized and, as a result, an inappropriately optimistic diagnosis may be given to the family.
6. The generalist should always be alert to the possibility of in-terfering issues such as psychosocial deprivation and/or unrec-ognized sensory deficits. When these issues are present as interfering factors, they tend to skew developmental findings in a pattern suggesting disproportionate delays in isolated areas of neurodevelopment. As most damage to the central ner-

vous system is diffuse in nature (e.g., hypoxic-ischemic injury), the results are expected to be diffuse. When peculiar patterns of disproportionate delay in isolated areas of neurodevelopment appear to be present, the generalist should look for interfering issues like psychosocial deprivation and/or unrecognized sensory deficits.

DEVELOPMENTAL DISABILITIES/ NEURODEVELOPMENTAL PRINCIPLES

As the generalist begins to interpret information gleaned through the neurodevelopmental history and examination, certain basic principles will help in organization and interpretation. Employment of these principles in organization and interpretation should enhance individual professional's understanding of developmental disabilities.

Many of our basic neurodevelopmental principles in developmental disabilities derive from our definition of developmental disabilities as chronic, neurologically based disabling conditions. Inherent in our definition of developmental disabilities is the understanding that central nervous system damage or dysfunction is common to all developmental disabilities, and, because of the irreversibility of such damage, developmental disabilities are understood to be chronic conditions that affect individuals across their lifespan. Throughout this text we will refer to developmental disorders that derive from central nervous system damage or dysfunction as primary (neurologically based) disabling conditions. Other neurodevelopmental principles include the concepts of secondary (derivative of primary) disabling conditions, associated deficits, dissociation of developmental dysfunction, and patterns of developmental delay deriving from static, progressive, and acute encephalopathies.

Primary (Neurologically Based) Disabling Conditions

Primary (neurologically based) disabling conditions reflect some form of central neurologic damage, brain pathology, or organic cerebral deficit. The primary disabling conditions most often seen in children and referred to in subsequent chapters include the following.

Cerebral Palsy

Cerebral palsy is a descriptive term (not a diagnosis) that means no more than that an affected child manifests significant deviation from the course of normal motor development. The incidence of cerebral palsy is 0.2%, contrasted with 3% for mental retardation. One might reasonably ask why the incidence of motor problems would be so much lower than that observed for mental dysfunction. The discrepancy in incidence figures for cerebral palsy versus mental retardation probably is explained in part by our inherent inability to detect subtle (but still clinically significant) levels of motor as opposed to cognitive dysfunction.

Mental Retardation

Mental retardation, like cerebral palsy, is a descriptive term that means no more than that an affected child manifests significant deviation from the course of normal mental and adaptive development. Specifically, this term is used when the intelligence quotient (IQ) and adaptive behavior quotient are more than two standard deviations below the mean for age on the test instrument used. As most tests have a mean of 100 and a standard deviation of 15 points, intelligence and adaptive quotients below 70 establish mental retardation.

Communication Disorders

The child with a communication disorder manifests a delay in connected language understanding and usage. Language dysfunction can occur in settings in which there is diffuse cognitive dysfunction, meaning that the disability in language is accompanied by a corresponding degree of perceptual dysfunction, and also in settings in which the major ob-served cognitive deficit appears to occur primarily in the language sphere, with relative sparing of visual perceptual function. When language dysfunction is accompanied by a corresponding degree of visual perceptual dysfunction, we refer to the language disability as occurring within a setting of mental retardation. Here there is no disproportionate disability (deviancy) in language and the child is simply slow in cognitive function, including language. When there occurs a disproportionate delay in language development compared with visual perceptual development, one begins to encounter certain oddities or peculiarities of behavior. Behavioral variations noted in children with disproportionate delays in language function compared with visual perceptual function include:

1. *Inconsistent eye contact.* When confronted verbally, the child typically exhibits only brief eye contact. The child may look about the room, fixing only briefly on visual objects of interest.

2. *Differential in auditory and visual attention span.* The child with discrepant language dysfunction may tend to ignore auditory stimuli, especially when visually occupied. The child will behave as if a hearing problem exists, but audiologic assessment will convey normal hearing with a failure to attend to auditory stimuli.

3. *Tendency to perseverate on visual problem-solving items.* The child will exhibit inordinate fascination or fixation on tasks tapping visual perception and problem solving. The child will have difficulty shifting from one such task to another.

4. *Exhibition of increasing frustration when confronted verbally.* The child with discrepant language dysfunction will exhibit frustration when confronted verbally and may avoid language confrontational situations.

What is obvious from this list of behaviors observed in children with discrepant language function (compared with visual perceptual abilities) is that many of these same behaviors are observed in children with infantile autism. In this disorder, the child exhibits "odd" or "peculiar" behavior (American Psychiatric Association, 1987) characterized by detachment and acts as if in his or her own world. In general, it can be said that all autistic children will be communicatively disordered in the sense that connected language understanding will be disproportionately delayed compared with other aspects of cognitive development. Similarly, all communicatively disordered children will have some autistic-like behaviors. However, not all communicatively disordered children will have enough autistic-like behaviors (i.e., be far enough along the autistic number line or rating scale) to be labeled as "autistic." The essence of being autistic is to be communicatively disordered, in the sense that language development is disproportionately delayed relative to visual perceptual development.

Learning Disabilities

Learning disabilities, compared with the other primary disabling conditions we have so far discussed, lie at the mild end of the developmental disabilities spectrum. We limit the use of the term learning disabilities to a condition in which an individual's academic achievement level is significantly below the level that would be predicted from the level of intellectual ability (Brown et al., 1992). The cause for the discrepancy between academic achievement and intellectual ability is presumed to be neurologically based. Although learning disabilities can occur concomitantly with other limiting conditions or environmental influences, they are not the direct result of these conditions or influences. Learning disabilities can occur in listening, speaking, reading, writing, reasoning, or mathematical abilities.

Attention-Deficit Hyperactivity Disorder (ADHD)

We follow criteria of definition as set forth in the *Diagnostic and Statistical Manual of Mental Disorders (DSM-III-R)* (Third Edition-Revised) of the American Psychiatric Association (1987). To be diagnosed as having attention-deficit hyperactivity disorder (ADHD), a child must meet criteria for developmentally inappropriate degrees of inattention (e.g., failure to finish things the youngster starts, failure to listen, easy distractibility, difficulty in concentrating or sticking to a play activity), criteria for impulsivity (e.g., acting before thinking, shifting from one activity to another, difficulty in organization, need for supervision, frequent calling out in class, and difficulty awaiting turns), and exhibit hyperactivity (e.g., run or climb excessively, have difficulty sitting still or staying seated). A distinction and separation of the issues of attention deficit disorder and hyperactivity (excessive motor activity) was indicated more clearly in the earlier version of the *Diagnostic and Statistical Manual of Mental Disorders-III (DSM-III)* (American Psychiatric Association, 1980), in that attention deficit disorder was described as occurring in the presence or absence of hyperactivity. The separation of these issues is obscured in the current term, attention-deficit hyperactivity disorder, but despite these reservations we will adhere throughout the text to the current terminology of attention-deficit hyperactivity disorder (ADHD).

Minimal Brain Dysfunction (MBD)

We will use this term in our text to refer to the child who has subtle and complex mixtures of cognitive and motor dysfunction. Components of MBD may include learning disabilities, language disabilities, other inconsistencies among various cognitive functions, ADHD, gross-, fine-, and oral-motor dyscoordinations. We conceptualize ADHD as part of a larger syndrome that was originally termed MBD. Throughout this text we will refer to the most common pattern of developmental delay in which the child exhibits complex mixtures of subtle neurological dysfunction—in these circumstances we are essentially referring to this older conceptualization of MBD.

Patterns of Primary (Neurologically Based) Disabling Conditions

As shown in Figure 1–2, there are at least three major patterns of primary damage to the nervous system. One of these patterns of developmental delay (Figure 1–2[b]) is that of the so-called "*static encephalopathy.*" This is an unfortunate term in the sense that it implies that development is somehow failing to progress, when, in actuality, development is progressing at a constant, although slower than normal rate. This course of developmental delay is illustrated by a diminished slope in Figure 1–2.

A second pattern of developmental delay illustrated in Figure 1–2[c] is that in which there is a falloff in rate of development at some point, with progressive deterioration over time and eventual frank regression in developmental function. This pattern is termed a "*neurodegenerative,*" or "*progressive encephalopathy,*" and is the pattern observed in ongoing insults to the central nervous system as might occur in inherited metabolic (and neurodegenerative) disorders.

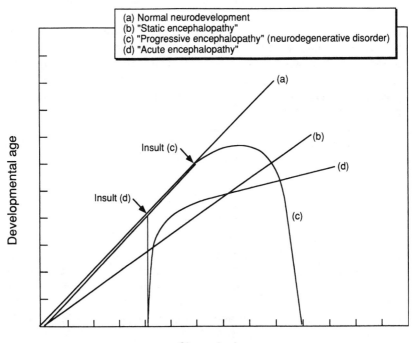

FIGURE 1–2. Patterns of developmental delay.

The final pattern of developmental delay is that resulting from acute insults to the central nervous system. In such an *"acute encephalopathy"* an abrupt falloff in development occurs at the onset of the acute insult, and this decline is followed by a rapid recovery and eventual establishment of a new rate of development that may or may not be the same as that observed before the insult (Figure 1–2[d]). Acute encephalopathies might result from such events as infection of the central nervous system, traumatic head injury, near drowning, and the like.

Secondary (Derivative of Primary) Disabling Conditions

Besides recognizing the presence of primary (neurologically based) disabling conditions in the individual with developmental disabilities, the generalist needs also to be aware of intercurrent *secondary (derivative of primary) disabling conditions.* Unlike the primary disabling conditions described previously, secondary disabling conditions do not have a direct neurological basis. They are, instead, the result of the primary disabling conditions, especially when the primary disabling conditions have not been properly managed. The most common secondary disabling conditions are poor self-concept and inappropriate attention-seeking behaviors. In addition to these two common secondary disabling conditions, children with primary neurological deficits may also exhibit such secondary characteristics as poor peer relationships, compliance problems, oppositional behaviors, depression, school phobia, and other problems of adjustment. It is obvious that all of these secondary behavioral and emotional disabling conditions need to be understood within the context of the family and parental perceptions of the vulnerability of their affected child.

Associated Deficits

Research has shown that approximately one-third of the individuals with developmental disabilities will exhibit a limitation in one of these areas of development, another third disabilities in two areas of development, and the remaining third disabilities in three or more areas of development (Conley, 1973). The more severe the disability is in any one area of developmental function, the greater the probability of disabilities in other areas. All of this translates into one of our most important neurodevelopmental principles pervading this text, namely, that individuals with neurodevelopmental delay are most apt to manifest deficits of development in *more than* one area of developmental function.

Generalists can bring focus on the issue of multiple disabilities through the concept of *associated deficits*. This term implies that although delays in one area of development appear most prominent, professionals examining children should be on the lookout for associated and perhaps more subtle areas of intercurrent developmental delay. In other terms, individuals with an obvious disabling condition can be anticipated, until proven otherwise, to exhibit associated deficits in other areas of developmental function—multiple disabilities, as opposed to isolated singular deficits, will predominate.

As a corollary to the idea of associated deficits, it is important to appreciate that it will sometimes be helpful diagnostically and therapeutically to *dissociate* inability to perform a particular task into its component parts—that is, to decide to what extent an individual's inability to perform a task stems from disability in one area of development as opposed to another. For example, when a child is asked to perform a task such as tying his or her shoe laces, satisfactory accomplishment depends on a combination of ability to visually conceptualize the task as well as the fine motor coordination to manipulate the objects. Failure to perform such a task could stem from maldevelopment in either the visual perceptual and/or fine motor area. By carefully observing a child's performance on such a task, the generalist can "dissociate" the process into its motor and perceptual components to decide the extent to which perceptual as opposed to motor deficits interfere with successful completion of the task.

Extent of Neurological Involvement

Besides associated deficits and the need to dissociate dysfunction into component motor and cognitive components, the other major issue the generalist needs to appreciate with individuals with developmental disabilities is that, in terms of extent of neurological involvement, mild degrees of disabilities predominate over more severe involvements. For example, the global statistic of 3% mental retardation conceals a skewed distribution. Most mentally retarded individuals (80%) function in a mildly retarded range. This same pattern of severity of disabling conditions applies to other areas of neurodevelopmental dysfunction—that is, in all spheres of dysfunction, mild disabilities prevail over more severe deficits. Some of these more subtle associated deficits, for example mild but functionally significant degrees of gross, fine, or oral motor dysfunction, may be overlooked unless the clinician has a high index of suspicion.

These findings of predominant associated deficits and mild degrees of involvement for individuals with neurodevelopmental disabilities can be better understood by realizing that disabilities like mental retardation and cerebral palsy derive from brain damage—that is, they are primary (neurologically based) disabling conditions. As most brain damage stems from diffuse insults to the nervous system, such as hypoxic-ischemic injury, it is reasonable to assume that developmental disabilities deriving from these insults will similarly be diffuse. Diffuse insults will most typically manifest as a pattern of associated deficits (multiple disabilities). Again, because mild insults may be anticipated to predominate, the associated deficits will most typically be of mild degree.

CONCLUSION

In this chapter we have introduced some neurodevelopmental principles that we believe underlie a generalist's approach to developmental disabilities. These include the concepts of primary (neurologically based) and secondary (derivative of primary) disabling conditions, associated deficits, and the spectrum of primary disabling conditions. We have indicated the need for a generalist to serve this population, to look for associated deficits and to dissociate dysfunction into its component parts. To become a generalist, one must expand perspective and skills to employ a neurodevelopmental history and examination as described in this chapter.

In subsequent chapters we present the primary neurologically based disabling conditions in more detail. For clarity, the primary neurologically based disabling conditions are initially presented as isolated aspects of dysfunction, but always with the ultimate understanding that dysfunction within one domain will need to be associated and interrelated with other areas of dysfunction. Additionally, we discuss the need for the generalist to be knowledgeable in secondary, behavioral, and emotionally based problems of children and families.

CHAPTER 2

CHILDREN WITH MOTOR IMPAIRMENT

Jean A. Patz, M.S., OTR
James Miedaner, M.S., PT

In the introductory chapter we defined developmental disabilities as chronic, neurologically based disabling conditions and emphasized that children with developmental disabilities will typically have primary neurologically based delays in more than one developmental domain. The role of the generalist in identifying primary neurologically based, as well as associated secondary behavioral and emotional problems, was presented in the form of the neurodevelopmental history and examination. In this chapter we look at how one of these primary neurologically based impairments, motor dysfunction, may manifest and be identified.

Motor dysfunction will be presented as derivative of damage in three areas of the brain: the motor cortex and upper motor neuron, the basal ganglia, and the cerebellum. Damage in these areas results in abnormalities in muscle tone, extraneous movements, and dyscoordination. For clarity, we initially present the motor dysfunction that derives from these three areas of the brain as discrete entities. In subsequent chapters we return to the concept of motor dysfunction admixed with other primary and secondary disabling conditions.

PATTERNS OF NORMAL MOTOR FUNCTION

Gross Motor Function

Gross motor development relates to large muscle control of posture and movements in prone (lying face down), supine (lying face up), rolling, sitting, crawling, standing, walking, and higher level motor and postural functions. The development of gross motor postures and movements appears to progress in an orderly and predictable sequence as shown in Table 2–1. As mentioned in Chapter 1, parents are usually very aware of gross motor developmental milestones and can usually tell the professional the level of their child's motor function. Some questions that can be used to obtain a developmental history from the parents and/or teacher concerning gross motor development are listed in Table 2–2.

Assessment of gross motor skills should include a quantitative and qualitative review. Several standardized tests exist for quantifying motor function and are listed in Table 2–3. None of these tests predict future outcome. They do afford an objective measure of motor performance and can serve to evaluate change over time.

Prone

When the full-term newborn is placed on the stomach, the child's arms and legs pull underneath the trunk in a tuck position. This reflects chronic flexed posturing from utero and inability to shift body weight to the stomach and legs. Shortly after birth, the full-term newborn can turn the head from side to side in this position, and by 3 to 4 months can rest on elbows, holding the head up to look around without falling. At approximately 6 to 7 months, the child can shift weight to one side and reach with the other arm. This ability to shift weight and maintain balance is critical to developing movement from one position to another and is a requisite motor strategy for higher levels of sitting, standing, and walking. At approximately 7 to 8 months, the child develops the ability to move from prone to a four-point position and subsequently to continue along the hierarchy of movement.

TABLE 2–1. Developmental motor milestones.

AGE	GROSS MOTOR	FINE MOTOR	ORAL MOTOR
1 mo		* hands fisted, grasp reflex * solitary play from 0 to 1 yr	* strong grasp on nipple with cupped tongue
2 mos	* lifts head in prone (face down)	* arms activate to object	
3 mos	* up onto forearms in prone	* swipes at objects/hands to midline * hands mostly open, grasp reflex diminishes	* sucks on spoon
4 mos	* up onto wrists in prone	* bilateral reach/contacts object * ulnar palmar grasp/shakes, pats, strikes	* introduce cup drinking between 4 to 6 mos
5 mos	* rolls over, supine to prone (face up to face down)	* reach in prone on forearms * palmar grasp on cube/transfer via mouth	* munching * one sip at a time from cup
6 mos	* sits without support * anterior propping in sitting	* circular reach in sitting with one arm * radial palmar on cube, raking grasp on pellet * direct transfer, mouths objects	* tongue and jaw quiets in anticipation of spoon
7 mos		* reach in prone on extended arms * inferior scissors grasp on pellet * release cube onto surface	* begins chewing with tongue lateralization
8 mos	* reaches to side in sitting * lateral propping in sitting	* direct reach in sitting with one arm * scissors grasp on pellet * clumsy release of cube into large opening	* handles junior/mashed food * uses upper lip to clear spoon
9 mos	* pulls to standing * crawl	* inferior pincer/pellet, radial digital/cube * controlled release of cube into large opening	* lateral lip seal on nipple * no liquid loss when sucking
10 mos		* 3-jawed chuck on cube, pincer on pellet * pokes	
12 mos	* walks independently * posterior propping in sitting	* direct reach in sitting/forearm supination * fine pincer on pellet, palmar grasp on crayon * precise release of cube/less finger extension * in/out play, throws, pulls, pushes, stacks	* handles coarsely chopped table food
14 mos		* tower of 2 cubes	* successful cup drinking (12-15 mos)
15 mos		* pincer with ulnar fingers stabilized * precise release of pellet into small container	* consecutive sips from cup
18 mos	* runs	* tower of 6 to 8 cubes * spontaneous scribble, imitates strokes	* handles meats and raw vegetables
2-3 yrs	* walks up stairs ("marking time")	* midline crossing is well established * parallel play 2 to 3 yrs, throws, cuts, fills, threads, rolls, pounds, squeezes, builds	* tongue movements across midline when chewing * jaw stability/cup drinking
3-4 yrs	* pedals tricycle * walks up stairs alternating feet and downstairs ("marking time")	* begins adult grasp on spoon * associative play 3 to 4 yrs, cuts, laces, sorts	
4-5 yrs	* balances on one foot by 4.5 yrs	* definite hand preference * transitional grasp on pencil (i.e., static tripod) * cooperative play, complex building, role play	
5-6 & up	* rides two-wheeled bicycle without training wheels	* precise grasp on pencil (i.e., dynamic tripod) * cooperative play, ties shoes, traces, copies	

Milestones compiled from Bledsoe & Shepherd (1982), Erhardt (1994), Folio & Fewell (1983), Knox (1974), and Morris & Klein (1987).

TABLE 2–2. Gross motor questionnaire for parents.

Age	Gross Motor Questions for Parents	Expectations
3-6 mo	Can they lift their head and look around while on their stomach?	Yes. Key is their ability to turn head from side to side.
	Is the head steady when you are carrying him/her?	Yes. Shouldn't wobble.
	Is diapering difficult?	No. Legs should be easily separated.
	In what position/s are arms and legs usually when lying on stomach/back?	Don't really know. Positions should vary. 1 or 2 positions suggest abnormal dominance of those postures.
6-12 mo	Can child bring feet to mouth, touch feet while lying on back?	Yes
	Does the child do a lot of kicking?	Yes
	How does the child move on the floor?	Tummy crawl or creep. No reports of stiff legs or very wide base of support
	Can the child sit and play with toys (reach for toys) without falling?	Yes. Especially 8-10 months. And to the sides as well as forward.
	Can the child get into and out of sitting on their own without crashing?	Yes. Around 8-10 months.
	Do they prefer one side or tend to lean to one side?	No. Predominance of asymmetrical postures indicative of decreased motor control, especially if seen >50% of the time.
12-24 mo	How often do they pull up to stand at the furniture?	Too many times to count. <10-15x per day is reason for concern.
	While standing (with or without support) can they reach down and pick up a toy?	Yes. Inability suggests instability and decreased motor control. (Seen frequently with hypotonia).
	How long have they been pulling up to stand?	Serves as possible bench mark for ambulation. Projections.
	When did he/she take first steps?	Bench mark for projecting additional upright skills. Acquisition. (Hopping, running, etc.)

Compiled by Jim Miedaner, MS, PT

TABLE 2–3. Selected pediatric assessment tools.

PURPOSE	SELECTED PEDIATRIC TESTS	AGE RANGE	AUTHOR	DATE
Development	Brigance Diagnostic Inventory of Early Development	0 to 7 yrs	Brigance	1978
Development	Developmental Programming for Infants/Young Children	0 to 35 mos	Schafer & Moersch (Eds.)	1981
Development	Hawaii Early Learning Profile	0 to 36 mos	Furuno, et al.	1990
Development	Learning Accomplishment Profile-Diagnostic Std. Assess.	2 1/2 to 6 yrs	Nehring, Nehring, Bruni, & Randolph	1992
Development	Vulpe Assessment Battery	0 to 5 yrs	Vulpe [being revised]	1977
Fine Motor	Erhardt Developmental Prehension Assessment (EDPA)	0 to 15 mos/1 to 6 yrs	Erhardt	1994
Fine/Gross Motor	Bayley Scales of Infant Development (Motor Scale)	1 to 42 mos	Bayley	1993
Fine/Gross Motor	Bruininks-Oseretsky Test of Motor Proficiency	4 1/2 yrs to 14 1/2 yrs	Bruininks	1978
Fine/Gross Motor	Peabody Developmental Motor Scales	0 to 83 mos	Folio & Fewell	1983
Handwriting	Children's Handwriting Eval. Scale for Manuscript Writing	1st & 2nd grades	Phelps & Stempel	1987
Handwriting	Children's Handwriting Evaluation Scale (cursive)	3rd thru 8th grades	Phelps, Stempel, & Speck	1984
Handwriting	Diagnosis and Remediation of Handwriting Problems	2nd grade and up	Stott, Moyes, & Henderson	1985
Handwriting	Test of Legible Handwriting (TOLH)	7 to 17 yrs	Larsen & Hammill	1989
Handwriting	Observations of Hand Skill of the "K & 1" Child	kindergarten & 1st grade	Benbow	1993
Handwriting	Observations for Cursive Handwriting Skills Training	3rd grade & up	Benbow	1993
Ocular Motor	Erhardt Developmental Vision Assessment (EDVA)	all ages	Erhardt	1989
Oral Motor	Multidisciplinary Feeding Profile	children	Kenny, et al.	1989
Oral Motor	Oral Motor Feeding Rating Scale	not stated	Jelm	1990
Oral Motor	Pre-Speech Assessment Scale	0 to 2 yrs	Morris	1982
Oral Motor/Sucking	Clinical Feeding Evaluation of Infants	newborns, infants	Wolf & Glass	1992
Quality of Movement	Evaluating Movement & Posture Disorganization	5 yr & above	Magrun	1989
Screen/Gross Motor	Milani Comparetti Motor Development Screening	0 to 2 yrs	Stuber, Dehne, Mielaner, & Romero	1987
Screen/Infant Motor	Movement Assessment of Infants	0 to 12 mos	Chandler, Andrews, & Swanson	1980
Screen/Neurological	Quick Neurological Screening Test	5 yrs & up	Mutti, Spalding, & Sterling	1978
Clinical Observations	Guide to Testing Clinical Observations in Kindergartners	5 to 6 1/2 yrs	Dunn	1981
SI/Sensory Integration	Sensory Integration and Praxis Tests	4 to 8 yrs, 11 mos	Ayres	1989
SI/Sensory Processing	Test of Sensory Functions in Infants	4 mos to 18 mos	DeGangi & Greenspan	1989
SI/Vestibular Based	DeGangi-Berk Test of Sensory Integration	3 to 5 yrs	DeGangi & Berk	1983
Visual Motor	Developmental Test of Visual-Motor Integration	2 to 15 yrs	Beery	1989
Visual Motor	Test of Visual Motor Integration	2 to 13 yrs	Gardner	1986
Visual Perception	Motor Free Visual Perception Test	4 to 8 yrs	Colarusso & Hammill	1972
Visual Perception	Test of Visual-Perceptual Skills	4 to 12 yr, 11 mos	Gardner	1982

Compiled by Jean A. Patz, MS, OTR/L

Supine

The full-term newborn lacks the strength and control to lift arms, legs, and head against gravity. The typical newborn posture in supine is one in which the arms are flat and slightly turned out, legs slightly bent and turned out, and head to one side or the other. By 3 to 4 months the child will show increased kicking, hand-to-mouth activities, and head balanced in the middle of the trunk. Hands will reach to the middle, but the child will have difficulty lifting hands or reaching. Hand-to-foot, foot-to-mouth, kicking and holding legs completely off the floor, are motor activities that become obvious by 5 to 7 months. By 6 to 7 months the child will initiate rolling from back to stomach. Sitting straight up from a supine posture will not occur until 3 to 4 years of age, when abdominal muscles are strong enough to accomplish this task.

Sitting

During the first 2 to 3 months, the full-term newborn develops increasing control of the head, neck, and upper trunk as preparation for sitting. Initial sitting attempts are characterized through support with both arms (anterior propping response) at approximately 5 to 6 months of age. By 6 to 7 months, a child can sit unsupported and by 8 months can reach to the side without falling (lateral protective or propping response). Sitting also requires an ability to posturally act, adjust, and respond to maintain a sitting balance. The final evolution of sitting (approximately 12 months) is the development of ability to protect oneself from a rearward fall by thrusting the arms backwards (posterior protective response). It should be noted that final refinement of sitting skills is still evolving at a time when other gross motor skills, such as independent walking, are intercurrently developing.

Standing

To maintain the standing position requires little strength, as the skeleton provides support necessary for standing. However, moving into a standing position requires strength typically not developed until 8 to 10 months of age. The child must be able to pull one leg forward while the opposite hip and trunk stay straight and then shift weight forward onto the leg. For the child who has developed the ability to pull to stand, cruising (meaning ambulation while holding onto objects, e.g., low table tops) is an antecedent to independent walking.

Walking

Taking a step from the standing position requires balance and the ability to shift weight from side to side. From the time the child first pulls to stand (8 to 10 months) to the time the child walks independently (11 to 14 months), the child practices stepping, weight shifting, and squatting, thus increasing leg strength and control. Walking is initially characterized by widely spread legs, short quick steps, and arms out for balance. With practice the arms come down, legs move closer together, and steps become longer. Independent ambulation is a significant milestone that parents and families anxiously await. As noted in Chapter 1, it is a milestone that most parents can accurately report.

Moving In and Out of Positions (Transitions)

Quite often when analyzing motor development there is a tendency to focus on postures to the exclusion of recognition of transitions between postures (movements). Because many children with delays of motor development have problems affecting transitions, it is critical that the generalist realize the importance of transitions to motor function. To move from one posture to another (e.g., sitting to four-point) requires the ability to shift weight, balance, use turning movements, and control speed of movements. Moving out of positions typically requires less refined control than moving into the same positions.

Fine Motor Function

Fine motor function relates to upper extremity capacities of reach, grasp, release, manipulation, bilateral control, and in-hand manipulation. The typical course of development of fine motor skills is outlined in Table 2–1. Some questions that can be used to obtain a developmental history from the parents and/or teacher concerning fine motor development are listed in Table 2–4. Referral is based on a number of concerns, rather than an isolated finding. As with gross motor development, several norm-referenced and criterion-referenced tests exist for quantifying or measuring fine motor function, although again, none predict future outcome. Selected instruments are presented in outline form in Table 2–3.

TABLE 2-4. Fine motor questionnaire for parents.

Age	Fine Motor Questions for Parents	Expectations/Approximate Ages
0-6 mo	Are your child's hands mostly open or fisted ? If open, at what age did this occur?	Hands are generally open most of the time by 3 mo. as the grasp reflex diminishes. Red flag-continual/strong fisting of hands with thumb in palm.
	Can your child bring his/her hands together in the middle of body?	Child can bring hands together by approximately 3-4 mo. Red flag-retracted arms, unable to meet in midline.
	Can your child push up on fully stretched (extended) arms when on their stomach?	Weight bear on forearms 3-4 mo., extended arms by 5 mo. Red flag-intolerance of prone position, cry whenever placed on stomach. Winging of scapulae.
	Can your child reach for a toy? If yes, at what age did this occur?	Swipe at an object by 3 mo., contact by 4 mo., and reach directly by 8 mo. Red flag-inability or lack of interest in any reaching after 6-8 mo.
6-12 mo	Can your child sit by himself/herself for play? If yes, when did this occur?	Independent sitting without use of arms occurs by 8 mo. Red flag-child relies on arms to sit vs. play. Parent reports use of pillows in sitting beyond 8-12 mo.
	Can your child transfer a toy from one hand to the other? When did this occur?	Indirect transfer via the mouth is followed by direct hand to hand transfer by 6-7 mo. Red flag-difficulty bringing two hands together or the inability to actively open hand for release.
	How does your child pick up a small object such as a small block?	Ulnar palmar grasp 4-5 mo., palmar 5 mo., radial palmar 6-7 mo., & radial digital 8-9 mo. Red flag-persistence of a primitive palmar grasp indicating lack of finger isolation.
	Can your child point/poke with the index finger?	Isolation of index finger occurs by 10 mo. Red flag-parent indicates that the child cannot point for communication or poke with the index finger.
	Does your child dislike touching certain textures?	Children are generally tolerant of various textures at any age. Red flag-extreme fussiness when touching objects/avoids or refuses to pick up age appropriate toys
12-24 mo	How does your child pick up a small object such as a pellet?	Pincer grasp begins by 9 mo. and is generally mature by 12 mo. Red flag-parent indicates that child has difficulty picking up small objects, rakes object.

TABLE 2–4 *(continued)*

	Which hand does your child use the most to reach for objects?	Hand preference begins to emerge after 12 mo. Either hand is used under one year. Red flag-strong hand preference reported under one year of age.
	Does your child have any problems letting go/releasing objects?	Precise release of a block into a small opening occurs by 12 mo., pellet by 15 mo., 2 block tower by 14 mo. Red flag-excessive dropping/or imprecise release.
	What can your child do with a crayon?	Imitation of scribbling occurs by 12-15 mo., scribble spontaneously by 18 mo. & imitation of lines by 2-2 1/2 yr. Red flag-persistent mouthing of crayon.
2-6 yrs.	Can your child reach across the middle of their body or do they tend to use the hand closest to the object?	Reaching across the midline of the body occurs by approximately 12 mo./well established by 2 yrs. Red flag-consistent use of the hand closest to the object without the ability to cross midline after 2 yrs.
	How does your child hold a spoon or fork?	Palmar grasp on spoon by 12-18 mo., adult grasp may occur by 3-4 yrs.
	What can your child do with an eating utensil?	Scoop with a spoon by 12-18 mo., stab with a fork by 3-4 yrs. Red flag-persistent finger feeding, refusal to use any utensils during preschool years.
	Is your child able to manipulate clothing fasteners (buttons, zipper, snaps)?	unzip by 18-24 mo, snap & unbutton by 2-3 yrs., small buttons by 4-5 yrs. Red flag-extreme difficulty learning how to do these activities, parent complains that it took "forever" to teach the child.
	Can your child use scissors at the same skill level as his/her classmates or peers?	variable-depends on exposure to scissors. snip with scissors by 2 yr., cut lines by 3 1/2 yrs., & cut well by 5 yrs. & up. Red flag- parent reports childs inability to coordinate holding & cutting after much instruction.
6 yrs. & up	Does your child have an awkward grasp on a pencil that seems different from classmates/peers? Please explain.	Mature grip on pencil (i.e. dynamic tri-pod mastered by 6 yrs. Red flag-thumb wraps over pencil, child reports hand cramps when writing, white knuckles during writing as child holds too tightly, weak or incoordinated grasp.
	Does your child consistently use one hand to manipulate utensils, scissors, etc.?	Consistent hand preference generally set before first grade. Red flag-parent can't tell handedness as child switches.

TABLE 2–4 *(continued)*

Does your child have any difficulty with handwriting-printing or cursive?	Printing is usually formally taught in kindergarten & 1st grade. Cursive in 2nd & 3rd. Red flag-teacher concerns: sloppy, illegible, poor spacing, presses too hard/tears paper, difficulty copying.
Can your child maintain upright sitting when writing?	Red flags-slumped posture, slides/falls out of chair, head held too close to paper holds head with hand, can't sit still.
Does your child hold the paper down when writing?	By 1st grade, child can stabilize paper adequately with the nondominant hand. Red flag-paper moves too much/ child doesn't attempt to hold paper.

Compiled by Jean Patz, MS, OTR; milestones from Erhardt 1994, Folio/Fewell 1983, and Stilwell 1987.

Reach

Reach typically progresses from asymmetrical movements, to bilateral movements (indicating development of symmetry), to unilateral movement where the child is able to differentiate one arm from the other. Arm movements during reach develop from flexion to gradual extension of the arm, wrist, and fingers and from pronation to supination of the forearm. Reach in the prone position develops in three planes, first prone on the floor, then up on forearms, followed by reaching on extended arms (Erhardt, 1994). An infant lying on the floor will free the arm for reach by shifting weight through the trunk. Initial attempts to reach on forearms results in collapse of the weight-bearing arm; successful reaching occurs at approximately 6 months. Reach on extended arms occurs by 7 to 8 months, when the child is able to stabilize the pelvic region, making lateral weight shift on extended arms possible. Random swiping, the first stage of reach in the supine position, occurs by 3 months and refines into more purposeful bilateral reach by approximately 4 to 5 months as the influence of primitive reflexes diminish and midline control emerges. Reach in sitting progresses from an immature circumducted two-handed approach to a more direct one-handed approach by approximately 8 months, with forearm supination occuring by approximately 12 months (Erhardt, 1994). With increasing postural control and development of hand preference, the child can reach beyond immediate boundaries and across the midline.

Grasp

Children use a variety of grasp patterns when manipulating the same object or objects of different shapes and sizes. Use of an exclusive, single grasp pattern would be considered atypical. Volitional grasp progresses from the ulnar (little finger) to the radial (thumb) side of the hand, from the palmar aspect of the hand to the digits, from flexion of the wrist to slight extension for stability, and from straight to rotational movements of the proximal joints of the thumb and radial fingers for opposition.

Erhardt (1994) describes the developmental sequence of grasp patterns on a cube and pellet. For grasp of large objects (e.g., a block), a whole hand (palmar) grasp emerges about 5 months of age. Initial grasp of smaller objects (e.g., a pellet) begins at 6 months, with raking maneuvers employing all the fingers except the thumb. The grasp for both large and small objects then evolves from the ulnar aspect, through the midline of the hand toward the radial side, with thumb and opposing fingers on a cube or pellet occurring by 9 to 10 months. Opposition is apparent as development of rotation occurs within the proximal joint of the thumb and index finger. By 12 months of age a child generally has sufficient fine motor control to grasp a small object such as a pellet by using the thumb and tip of the index finger with flexion of the 4th and 5th digits and active wrist extension (fine pincer).

Grasp on a writing tool progresses from immature/primitive palmar grasps in which the arm moves as a unit to static, transitional grasp patterns using hand movements initiated at the wrist and finally to precision grasps requiring finely coordinated movements of the forefingers and thumb; type of task and sex of the child account for variation along this continuum (Schneck & Henderson, 1990). Children use less mature grips for coloring tasks that require gross movements while using mature grips for drawing or writing tasks that require finer movements; girls tend to use more mature grips than boys until age $4\frac{1}{2}$ with uniformity of grips occurring thereafter according to Schneck and Henderson. The static tripod is an example of a transitional grasp in which the grip pattern is similar to the dynamic tripod except that the hand moves as a unit (Rosenbloom & Horton, 1971). The dynamic tripod grasp (cf. Figure 2–1), one of the more common precise grasp patterns for handwriting, involves pad to pad opposition of the thumb and index finger with the pencil resting on the radial portion of the middle digit; a rounded open web space; slight wrist extension; flexion of the ulnar digits for stability; and precise, alternating flexion and extension movements of the digits (Long, Conrad, Hall, & Furler, 1970; Rosenbloom & Horton, 1971). Schneck and Henderson (1990) indicate that primitive grasp patterns are rarely seen over 4 years of age; transitional grasps typically occur between $4\frac{1}{2}$ and 6 years of age and mature grasps have been observed in children as young as 3 years, but are more typically seen in children $6\frac{1}{2}$ years and older.

Release

Voluntary release begins with nonselective dropping and then transfer of objects from hand to hand by 5 to 6 months of age (Erhardt, 1994). By 7 months, a child can release an object selectively against a surface. Release of a large object (a block) into a large container develops by 9 months and precise release into a small container by 12 months; release of a small object (pellet) into a small container occurs at 15 months (Erhardt, 1994). The child is able to begin graded release of objects (e.g., building a tower) by this age, as the foundational motor skills of shoulder, wrist, and finger stability occur with the ability to isolate partial forearm supination.

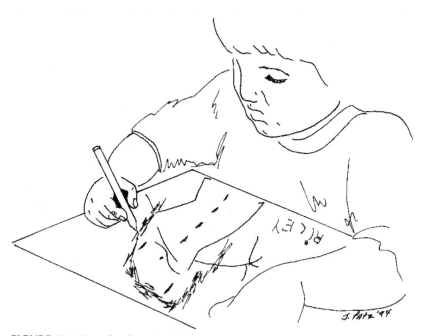

FIGURE 2–1. Preschool-aged child using a tripod grasp on a marker with wrist extension, thumb/finger opposition, open web space, flexion of ulnar digits, and partial forearm supination. Static grasp used when drawing or coloring may change to a dynamic grasp when printing.

Manipulation

Age-appropriate manipulation of toys, scissors, eating utensils, writing tools, and clothing fasteners requires a child to coordinate the fine motor foundational skills of reach, grasp, release, and bilateral development. Refinement of these skills continues throughout the school years as in-hand manipulation abilities mature.

Bilateral development progresses through the following stages: (1) asymmetrical unilateral movements; (2) bilateral movements which are first symmetrical and then alternating; (3) unilateral alternating movements; (4) bilateral opposing movements; and (5) refined unilateral control with development of a hand preference (Abell et al., 1978). A 2-month-old infant is motorically asymmetrical, as demonstrated by the asymmetrical tonic neck reflex and predominantly unilateral attempts at swiping. Bilateral development begins when the child can bring hands to the chest in midline by three months. Bilateral reaching occurs at 4 to 5 months, followed by bilateral object holding or transferring between hands at 6 to 8 months, and clapping hands or banging objects together at 8 to 12 months. Unilateral alternating movements occur between 12 and 24 months; either hand manipulates the object while the other hand assists, first passively in building a tower then actively in putting pop beads together. By approximately 24–36 months, the child is able to use bilateral opposing movements to tear paper. The manipulating hand becomes more predominant by approximately 3 years with a definitive hand preference occurring by kindergarten for tasks such as coloring, cutting with scissors, and eating with utensils.

In-hand manipulation described by Exner (1990, 1992) is the fine adjustment of objects within the hand, including translation (finger to palm and palm to finger), shift, and rotation (simple and complex). These skills primarily emerge after 1 year of age and show a heightened period of development from about 2 to 4 years (Exner, 1990). Translation is movement of an object in a linear fashion; moving a small object such as a coin from the fingers to the palm is easier than from the palm to the finger tips. Shift is a slight movement of an object with the object held at the thumb and finger pads; examples of this skill include shifting a pen up or down within the fingers, separating thin pieces of paper, or turning pages in a book. Moving an object in one hand around its axis is categorized as rotation; simple rotation involves partial rotation 90° or less (as in twisting off a cap), whereas complex rotation requires more extensive rotation between 180–360° (Exner, 1992). Separation of the ulnar and radial sides of the hand is a prerequisite for mature in-hand manipulation. This occurs when the child is able to stabilize objects with the ulnar fingers after manipulating them with the radial fingers of the same hand (such as picking up pennies one at a time and storing them under the 4th and 5th digits).

Oral Motor Function

Oral motor development relates to the tongue, jaw, lip, and cheek movements needed in sucking, swallowing, munching/chewing, spoon-feeding, and cup drinking. The typical course of development of oral motor skills is outlined in Table 2–1. Some questions that can be used in eliciting a history of development of oral motor function are listed in Table 2–5. Selected instruments for describing oral motor status are presented in Table 2–3.

Sucking

The immature suckling pattern is characterized by anterior-posterior tongue movements with wide jaw excursions and a loose lateral lip seal creating liquid loss; mature sucking involves vertical up and down tongue movements with smaller jaw gradations and lip closure creating suction (Morris & Klein, 1987). The infant feeds by wrapping the tongue around the nipple in a cupped configuration, channeling the liquid for swallow. The jaw provides stability and moves rhythmically with the tongue. By approximately 9 months of age, lateral lip seal has matured to the extent that the child no longer loses liquid when sucking (Morris & Klein, 1987). The rate of nonnutritive sucking with a pacifier is approximately two sucks per second with short bursts and pauses; in contrast nutritive sucking on a bottle is slower, at a rate of one suck per second with longer bursts of sucking and fewer rests (Wolff, 1968). A newborn generally has no difficulty initiating sucking when hungry (grasp on the nipple is strong) and can complete a bottle within 20–30 minutes (Morris & Klein, 1987).

Swallowing

Swallowing involves four distinct stages: oral preparatory, oral, pharyngeal, and esophageal (Logemann, 1983). Food and liquid are prepared for swallow in the oral preparatory phase. The oral phase begins when the tongue moves the prepared bolus of food or liquid to the back of the mouth into the pharynx. The pharyngeal phase starts with the triggering of the swallow reflex as the food or liquid moves through the pharynx. At the point of swallow, the child will stop breathing momentarily as the airway closes to prevent aspiration (Logemann, 1983). The final phase of swallowing involves the passage of food or liquid through the esophagus into the stomach.

TABLE 2–5. Oral motor questionnaire for parents.

Age	Oral Motor Questions	Expectations/Approximate Ages
0-6 mo	Is it difficult for you to hold your child on your lap or place them in an infant seat during meals?	Child's body generally molds to parent's arms or to a seat. Red flag-abnormal posture (too limp or stiff) or constant fussiness when held.
	Does your child have any swallowing problems?	Red flag - frequent coughing or choking during or after meal, wheezing or gurgly voice, delayed swallow, residual food in in mouth, or excessive liquid loss.
	Does your child have any history of pneumonia?	Red flag- history of aspiration pneumonia or report of previous swallow studies.
	Does your child have any difficulty initiating sucking from a bottle when hungry and alert?	Full term infant can generally initiate a suck easily when hungry. Red flag-persistent difficulty starting to suck, difficulty inserting nipple, constant biting on nipple.
	Have you needed to adjust the nipple in any way to make sucking easier for your child?	Red flag- report from the parent of cutting larger hole in the nipple to increase intake or difficulty finding a nipple that works consistently.
	Does your child have a strong grasp on the nipple?	When hungry & alert, an infant has a strong grasp on the nipple. Red flag-weak grasp, no suction on nipple, poor intake.
	Approximately how long does it take for your child to drink a full bottle when hungry?	A healthy infant can generally complete a bottle in 20-30 minutes when hungry and alert. Red flag-takes more than 40-60 min. on a consistent basis.
6-12 mo	Does your child seem to drool more than you would expect for his/her age? Is your child currently teething?	Teething generally occurs between 6-18 mo. with an increase in drooling. Red flag-persistent, excessive drooling beyond the teething phase, bib constantly soaked.
	Can your child hold own bottle?	Independent holding occurs by 6-9 mo.
	What type of food texture is your child currently eating?	Depending on culture & medical advice, strained/pureed food between 3 & 8 mo., junior/mashed food by 8 mo., coursely chopped regular food by 12 mo. Red flag-difficulty transitioning to regular food -persists on baby food beyond 12-15 mo.
	Can your child use their lips to clear food off a spoon or do you have to wipe spoon upwards to clear food?	Upper lip clearance on spoon begins by 7-8 mo. Red flag- parent has to consistently wipe spoon upward beyond 9-12 mo.

(continued)

TABLE 2-5 (continued)

	At what age did you introduce a cup to your child?	Introduction of the cup usually occurs by 5-6 mo. Red flag-repeated attempts to give cup fail; child cries or forcefully pushes the cup away.
	Can your child sit independently without using arms for support?	Independent sitting occurs by 6-8 mo. Red flag-child needs pillows for support beyond 8-12 mo.
12-18 mo	How well can your child drink from a cup?	Successful cup drinking occurs by 12-15 mo. Red flag-persistent cough, choking, dehydration, or excessive liquid loss.
	Can your child chew (grind up) regular table food?	Tongue lateralization begins by 7 mo., chewing occurs by 10-12 mo. Red flag-persists on baby food, food stays in front of mouth, choking/gagging, food loss.
All ages	Is feeding your child relaxing and enjoyable?	Feeding times are usually pleasant. Red flag-parent stressed/concerned about intake
	Does your child tolerate being fed by others?	Children will generally allow others to feed them except when experiencing stranger anxiety. Red flag-child will only tolerate eating from one individual; child cries or refuses to be fed by others on a consistent basis, parent is stressed due to no respite.
	Approximately how much time does it take for you to feed your child the largest meal of the day?	Red flag-feeding times that persist beyond 45-60 minutes when the child is alert and hungry/parent does not enjoy feeding child.
	Does your child have any behavior problems during mealtimes?	Red flag-picky eater, ongoing negative behaviors which may be related to oral motor dysfunction or aspiration/reflux.
	How does your child react to chunky/solid food?	Red flag-consistent negative reaction to presentation of solid foods beyond 12 mos. may indicate oral motor dysfunction, oral hypersensitivity, or developmental delay.

Compiled by Jean Patz, MS, OTR; milestones from Morris, Klein (1987) and Logemann (1983).

Munching/Chewing

Munching is an immature pattern of chewing in which the tongue is used to mash food against the palate. It consists of straight up and down tongue and jaw movements that typically emerge at 5 to 6 months. Development of tongue lateralization, rotary jaw movement, and lip use in chewing is outlined by Morris and Klein (1987). Tongue lateralization begins at approximately 7 months, with the tongue shifting from center to the side and progresses to include lateralization across the midline by 2 years of age. Diagonal rotary jaw movements emerge at about 5 to 6 months changing to circular rotary movements with food transfer across midline by 2 years. Lip use during chewing begins at 6 months, with tightening of the corner progressing to some contact of the middle or lateral borders of the lips by 9 months. The child begins to use lip closure to control the food by 15 months; by 2 years, food loss no longer occurs. Consistent lip closure may occur between 3–4 years, dependent on cultural expectations. The development of chewing with tongue lateralization allows the child to progress from cereals and strained foods to transitional foods such as junior, ground, or mashed table foods by approximately 8 to 9 months, coarsely chopped food by 12 months, and regular table food with meats and some raw vegetables by 18 months (Morris & Klein, 1987).

Spoon Feeding

Upper lip control, an essential requisite to clearing food from the spoon, typically begins around 8 months of age (Morris & Klein, 1987). Prior to the point of upper lip control, a child presented with food on a spoon will attempt sucking motions on the spoon. The parent must withdraw the spoon from the mouth in an upward fashion to clear the food. As the child develops better head control, jaw stability, and upper lip usage, this is no longer necessary, as the child can clear the food independently. Beyond 6 months, the tongue and jaw remain quiet in anticipation of the spoon (Morris & Klein, 1987).

Cup Drinking

Cup drinking is usually introduced between 4 and 6 months, with successful cup drinking accomplished by 12–15 months of age (Morris & Klein, 1987). A child typically initiates cup drinking using immature sucking patterns. Initially the child will only take one sip at a time and by approximately 1 year can accomplish consecutive swallowing. Consecutive swallowing may occur earlier, when drinking from a spouted cup versus a regular cup. Tongue movements progress from simple protrusion during the 1st year (which causes liquid loss) to tongue tip elevation by approximately 2 years of age (Morris & Klein, 1987). Jaw movements in drinking progress from wide up and down movements to smaller excursions. External jaw stability (biting on the cup rim) while drinking is usually seen in a child 18 months of age, maturing to internal jaw stability by 24 months (Morris & Klein, 1987).

PATTERNS OF MOTOR DYSFUNCTION/
TONAL DIFFICULTIES

Hypertonus

Hypertonus represents one extreme of a continuum of tonal abnormalities, ranging from markedly decreased (hypotonus) to markedly increased (hypertonus). Hypertonus is derivative of lesions of the upper motor neuron, cortical spinal tract, and/or motor areas of the cerebral cortex. Unless severe, hypertonus will not be obvious to parents or the generalist before 6 months of age. However, as the child with underlying hypertonus begins to attempt movement, certain patterns of abnormal posture and movement will be observed.

As shown in Figure 2–2, the child with hypertonus will tend to maintain the lower extremities in an extended and adducted (legs pulled together) posture, with the feet pointing down and turned in, the trunk tilted to the side, and the shoulders depressed and retracted. Below 6 months of age these postures may not be abnormal, unless they are present more than 50% of the time and interfere with the child's ability to perform other movements. Persistence of these postures after 7 months of age suggests motor delay and can put the hip joint at risk for dislocation.

The child with hypertonus exhibits a decreased ability to rotate the trunk and/or weight shift from side to side, significantly limiting ability to move in and out of sitting. In an attempt to maintain sitting, the child may engage in a variety of compensatory strategies including: head extension to maintain balance; holding onto objects to maintain stability; extension and adduction of the lower extremities to maintain balance; and/or retraction of the upper extremities to increase trunk stability and extension. For milder cases, these atypical postures may not be obvious until the child is asked to stand or move. Increasing task difficulty is an effective strategy for identifying milder tonal abnormalities. Analysis of transitions from one position to another is essential for recognizing mild hypertonus.

Additional deficiencies of movement and posture in children with hypertonus include a tendency to move the body and limbs as a total unit characterized by patterns of total flexion and/or extension. For example, when attempting to pull-to-stand, the child does so with both legs either completely stiff or completely flexed. A similar pattern is seen as the child attempts to crawl or creep, with movement characterized by strong upper extremity effort with resultant stiff extension or flexion of the lower extremities (bunny hopping). Sometimes hypertonus can create atypical sequences of motor development, as with a child

TYPICAL DEVELOPMENT	ATYPICAL - HYPERTONIA

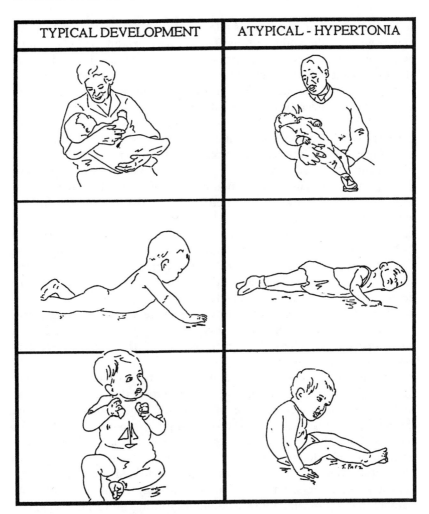

FIGURE 2-2. Atypical postures in children with hypertonus that interfere with activities such as being held, pushing up on arms, or reach in sitting.

who can stand but is unable to sit. Children can use atypical hypertonus through the head, trunk, upper and lower extremities to maintain a supported standing position, whereas the same distribution of hypertonus may preclude sitting.

Hypertonus in the upper extremities may produce the following atypical postures: elevated and/or retracted shoulders, protracted scapulae, adducted and internally rotated upper extremities, flexed elbows with pronated forearms, flexed wrists with ulnar deviation, and fisted hands with adducted thumbs. These atypical upper extremity postures can make it difficult for a child to bring hands to the midline, to reach fully, and/or to roll when in a supine (face up) posture. In prone (face down) posture, the child with hypertonus may exhibit patterns of total extension or total flexion and be restricted in weight bearing and weight shifting on the upper extremities. This, in turn, will affect the child's ability to reach in prone. Hypertonus in the arms, shoulders, and trunk can inhibit shoulder flexion needed for crawling.

Reach, grasp, and release may all be adversely affected by increased tone in the upper extremities. Increased tone in the elbow, wrist, and finger flexors interferes with reach and limits range and arm/hand placement. Increased tone in the forearm will pull the arm into a pronated posture, preventing supination needed for skilled fine motor tasks. The child's reach may be asymmetrical if the extremities have differential tone. Grasp will be inhibited by increased wrist flexion with ulnar deviation and by the thumb being drawn in toward the palm (Figure 2–3). These problems interfere with thumb and finger tip opposition needed to prehend small objects or maintain grasp on a pencil. The first stage of release, direct hand-to-hand transfer, will be inhibited by shoulder retraction, preventing the hands from meeting in the midline. Persistence of a primitive grasp reflex, or exaggerated wrist flexion and limited thumb extension due to hypertonia, may also interfere with controlled release. These children lack isolated finger movement necessary for in-hand manipulation.

In the oral motor area, thrusting of the tongue or jaw, retraction of the upper lip, or persistence of a tonic bite reflex may all arise as maladaptive functions because of increased tone. Abnormal tongue thrusting may manifest as pushing the nipple, spoon, or food out of the mouth and by poor quality chewing because of lack of tongue lateralization. The tongue appears thick and bunched, interfering with channeling food for swallowing or wrapping around the nipple for efficient sucking. Persistence of a tonic bite may be inferred from the parents' history of the child's involuntarily biting down on a spoon or nipple and its interference with putting a spoon in the child's mouth. Upper lip retraction can interfere with closure on the nipple, clearance of food from the spoon, and lip closure on the cup as the lips are pulled back. Additional indications of oral dysfunction stemming from hypertonus would be a history of excessively long feeding sessions, persistent dependence on bottle feeding or baby food (e.g., pureed, junior or ground), persistent drooling, and poor oral intake.

Hypotonus

Hypotonus (decreased motor tone) represents the other extreme (compared with hypertonus) of the continuum of total abnormalities. It can

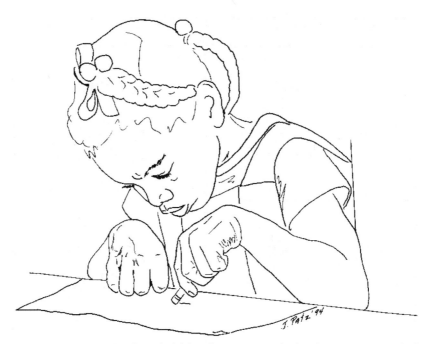

FIGURE 2–3. Preschool-aged child with spastic cerebral palsy using an atypical palmar grasp on a crayon; hypertonus interferes with drawing and stabilizing the paper. Note poor postural control, restricted arm movement, limited forearm supination, and wrist flexion with ulnar deviation.

be considered derivative of interruption of the connecting pathways between the cerebellum, cerebral cortex, brain stem, and spinal cord. In infancy, the parents describe the child with hypotonus as floppy or like a "rag doll." The generalist should monitor carefully any child who, as shown in Figure 2–4, presents with decreased spontaneous movement and/or excessive abduction and external rotation of the upper and lower extremities (arms and legs widely spread and turned out). Unless severe, it is difficult to definitively diagnose hypotonus before 4 months of age.

Beyond about 4 to 5 months of age, the child with hypotonus may exhibit reciprocal kicking of the lower extremities while in a supine (face up) posture, but will typically be unable to lift and bring the legs together. This decreased ability to control extremities against gravity will be demonstrated by an inability to perform feet-to-hands or feet-to-mouth activities. In the prone (face down) posture the child has limited ability to push onto extended arms, will maintain the arms in an extended and externally rotated posture, and, as a result, will have difficulty weight shifting from one side to the other for reaching, rolling,

TYPICAL DEVELOPMENT	ATYPICAL - HYPOTONIA

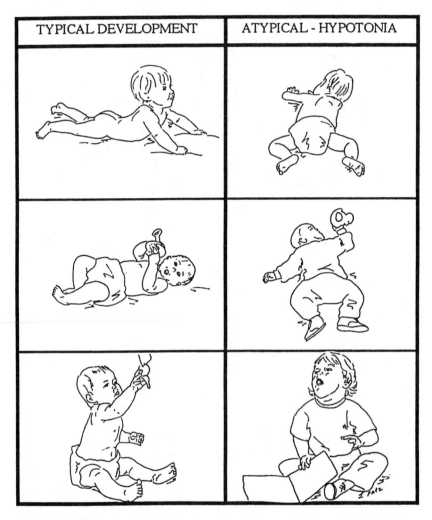

FIGURE 2-4. Poor antigravity postures in children with hypotonus that interfere with midline play skills and motor development.

and playing. The parents will interpret all of this as the child not liking to be on his or her stomach.

When attempting sitting, the child with hypotonus maintains a slumped posture, propping with the upper extremities. The arms and legs will be widely spread and externally rotated. The wide-based postures of both the upper and lower extremities interfere with weight shifting and ability to come in or out of the sitting position.

With regard to acquisition of walking skills, the child with mild to moderate hypotonus may take an extended period (up to 12 months longer than usual) to progress from cruising to independent walking. The child will attempt to gain increased stability in standing by widening the base and locking the knees in hyperextension.

Decreased tone in the upper extremities affects stability of the shoulder girdle limiting distal control for reach and grasp. Because of intercurrent hypotonus in the trunk and resultant instability in sitting, the child will tend to use the arms for supported sitting versus purposeful reaching and grasping. When the child with hypotonus attempts grasping, there is a tendency to persist with primitive grasp patterns such as the palmar grasp. Joint instabilities in the hands force the child to develop compensatory (atypical) patterns of grasp that lack precision and efficiency. An older child with hypotonia may hold a pencil tightly by wrapping the thumb around the pencil shaft; this compensatory stabilization posture may interfere with writing efficiency. Because of the delay in development of a more mature grasp, the child with hypotonus may demonstrate frequent dropping and a clumsy release for an extended period.

Hypotonus in the oral region frequently results in the child exhibiting an open mouth posture with subsequent drooling. This open mouth posture prevents adequate lip seal around a nipple, cup, or spoon and results in liquid or food loss. The hypotonic tongue will be flat rather than cupped, which interferes with sucking as the child cannot wrap the tongue around the nipple or channel the bolus for swallowing. The open mouth posture leads to difficulty initiating a suck. These children may persist in taking a bottle, as they have poor jaw stability and lip closure on the cup. Oral hypotonus additionally results in exaggerated and persistent tongue protrusion preventing progression to higher textured foods and interfering with adequate intake of food. Poor chewing in the child with hypotonus may derive from difficulties approximating and rotating the jaw, as well as poor tongue lateralization. The parents will report, and the therapist will observe, persistent drooling, inadequate lip closure, exaggerated tongue protrusion, and poor feeding patterns.

Mixed Tonal Abnormalities

In the discussion of hypertonus and hypotonus above, these extremes of the continuum of tonal abnormalities were presented as discrete entities. In actuality, most children with motor dysfunction will have mixtures of these tonal extremes operating, most probably with hypertonus and hypotonus admixed throughout the body.

A very common pattern of such mixed tonal abnormality is that in which the child exhibits hypertonus of the extremities with concurrent hypotonus throughout the trunk and neck. The child with this tonal distribution will posture with the extremities much as described for the child with hypertonus, but will simultaneously show poor head control, slumping postures with emerging sitting, and delays in acquisition of independent walking skills as reported for the child with hypotonus. The parents will report more complicated admixtures of postures and motor development than described for the "pure" instances of hypertonus and hypotonus. Upon examination, the child will be observed to have complicated admixtures of tone, posture, and degrees of motor development. This may manifest as atypical sequences of motor development with, for example, the child developing aspects of sitting before completion of prone development.

PATTERNS OF MOTOR DYSFUNCTION/ DYSCOORDINATION AND EXTRANEOUS MOVEMENTS

In our discussion of motor control so far, we have discussed aberrancies of muscle tone, either increased (hypertonus), decreased (hypotonus), or mixed, that would be seen and reported by the parents in the neurodevelopmental history or noted by an examiner as part of the neurodevelopmental examination. In this section we address two additional patterns of motor dysfunction, dyscoordination and extraneous movements, as well as describe expected patterns of complicated admixtures of these dysfunctions.

Dyscoordination

The cerebellum is an essential component of the central nervous system concerned with control or modulation of motor movement. In the section on hypotonus, the cerebellum was ascribed a role in the maintenance of normal muscle tone, and one manifestation of cerebellar dysfunction, hypotonus, was described. Besides this role in maintaining normal muscle tone, the cerebellum plays a role in the following aspects of muscle movement:

1. initiating and terminating volitional movement;
2. controlling direction of volitional movement;
3. grading velocity during movement;
4. controlling many-jointed movements;
5. controlling "automatic" continuous movements;

disorders of these aspects are termed *ataxia*.

The child with significant motor dysfunction stemming from the cerebellum can be expected to manifest disorders of posture and movement that we term hypotonic and/or ataxic "cerebral palsy." In the neurodevelopmental history, the parents will typically report that their child exhibits postural abnormalities, but no particular movement abnormalities as long as the child is lying in bed. The child with cerebellar dyscoordination can maintain postures such as sitting or standing, but may have trouble combining movement with other postures, such as reaching while sitting or taking a step from standing. The child with cerebellar dyscoordination has obvious tremor and unsteadiness when attempting movement. It is difficult for these children to "feel" how much to bend and straighten the leg, resulting in exaggerated leg movement in stepping.

Lesser degrees of cerebellar dyscoordination may only be obvious when the child attempts detailed activities with the hands during unsupported sitting. The child with combined problems of tonal control and cerebellar dyscoordination exhibits considerable joint instability and resultant difficulties with maintenance of posture and initiation of movement. In other words, children with cerebellar hypotonia and ataxia may present with similar observed abnormalities of posture and movement.

Extraneous Movements and Atypical Postures

When neurodevelopmentalists use the term movement disorders, they generally refer to extraneous movements characterized by dyscoordinated muscle contractions deriving from central nervous system dysfunction, but excluding the types of cerebellar dysfunction described above. Chorea and athetosis are examples of such extraneous movements. *Chorea*, derived from the Greek word for dance, consists of involuntary, quick jerking movements at rest. *Athetosis* is used to describe slow twisting, wormian-like movements.

The substrate for both chorea and athetosis is damage to part of the brain termed the basal ganglia. Within the basal ganglia there is normally a delicate balance of neurotransmitters requisite for appropriate communication. When this balance is upset, movement disorders may manifest. Besides playing a role in maintaining purposeful movement, the basal ganglia help in the maintenance of posture. The term *dystonia* refers to severely distorted postures of the trunk, neck, and that portion of the extremities closest to the trunk. These distorted postures can also, in part, be ascribed to damage to the basal ganglia.

The parents of a child with postural and movement disorder deriving from damage to the basal ganglia may report that their child exhibits complex mixtures of quick, jerky and slow, twisting motor movements, as well as severely distorted body postures. The child may have difficulty bearing weight on the upper extremities when placed face down (prone). Sitting postures vary from widely spread apart (abducted) to stiff and pulled together (extended and adducted) in an attempt to stabilize the body. Head and trunk are typically weak and/or floppy (hypotonic).

Parents will describe, and the examiner will observe, a child in a continual state of movement. Minimal control is noted in the midranges; the child has difficulty grading/controlling self movements. The child will attempt to minimize interference from involuntary movements by using compensatory stabilizing patterns. In attempting to maintain sitting postures, the child with athetosis may resort to holding on with hands, or locking their legs around the chair for external stability. There may be a poor quality reach, grasp, and release, with the child frequently missing the target and only effective in gaining stability when the arm is fully extended. The child will attempt to minimize interfering involuntary movements of the upper extremities by using primitive grasp patterns such as a palmar grasp for stabilization, elevating the shoulders for head stability, locking the elbows in hyperextension, and adducting and internally rotating the arms to assist in distal control. Visual tracking and eye/hand coordination may be impaired by involuntary head and eye movements.

Involuntary movements may also be observed in the mouth. Extraneous movements of the tongue, jaw, lips, and cheeks with compensatory stabilizing patterns, such as biting on the spoon or cup, may interfere with eating. There is a lack of proximal stability and midrange control needed for graded oral movements. Compared to the child with hypertonus, the child with athetosis may demonstrate a greater degree of tongue and jaw thrusting because of involuntary movements. The parents of an infant with involuntary movements of the mouth may report that they have difficulty inserting the nipple and that the child has difficulty sustaining contact with the nipple. Chewing is labored and incomplete because of the wide gradations of tongue and jaw movements. Active lip closure on the spoon may be delayed because of compensatory lip retraction used for stability. Cup drinking is affected, as the child has difficulty maintaining lip contact on the cup rim leading to liquid loss; extraneous tongue movements interfere with posterior transfer of liquid for swallowing.

MOTOR ASSESSMENT

Before the motor evaluation, the parent is contacted to have the child's favorite toys, familiar food and utensils, and any pertinent positioning equipment utilized at home available for the evaluation. For the oral motor assessment, the caregivers are requested to record their child's food and liquid intake for 3 consecutive days.

Necessary preassessment information is obtained from medical/ nutritional records including: diagnoses, medical and nutritional status, medications, and any information from previous gross/fine motor, play, oral motor, or swallowing evaluations. An interview is conducted with the primary caregivers, utilizing the questionnaires listed in Tables 2–2, 2–4, and 2–5, to obtain the child's developmental history as well as the parents' overall concerns.

The evaluation is scheduled at a time when the child is expected to be most alert, during a typical mealtime is preferable for the oral motor assessment. The evaluation materials needed include the actual test kit and forms, a variety of toys appropriate for the gross and fine motor portion, and food textures available for the oral motor assessment (baby food, dry cereal, raisins, dried fruits, etc.), as well as eating utensils. The optimum setting for testing is in the child's natural environment, if possible.

The actual assessment begins by observing the caregiver position the child. During the gross and fine motor assessment, the therapist evaluates existence of primitive postural reflexes, status of extremity range of motion and integrity, hypo-/hypersensitivity to touch, postural control of the child, and gross and fine motor abilities needed for functional independence in play, self-care tasks, or schoolwork. Typical and atypical movement components of vision may also be noted. The child's behavior and socialization during play are documented. Visual motor, visual perception, self-care, and sensory integration testing may also be conducted to rule out other contributing factors.

The oral motor assessment begins by observing the parent feed the child, noting positioning of the parent in relationship to the child, how the parent positions the child, method the caregiver uses to feed the child, and the interaction during eating. The food and liquid are measured before and after feeding to determine intake over time. The therapist feeds the child, noting: oral and postural tone, existing primitive oral and postural reflexes, positioning/postural status of the child, oral structures (palate, teeth, gums, frenulum, etc.), sensitivity in the oral region (hypo/hyper sensitivities), and typical and atypical movement components of the tongue, jaw, lips, and cheeks in the appropriate eating functions (sucking/swallowing, munching/biting/chewing, spoon feeding, and cup drinking). The child's overall behavior during meal/evaluation session is recorded. An occupational therapist may also assist in positioning and feeding the child during swallowing studies when indicated.

The initial evaluation report includes a summary of the quality of motor patterns, typical and atypical motor components, and a summary of the child's current developmental skill level. The child's strengths and weaknesses are compiled and a treatment plan is formulated when indicated. Information from interdisciplinary team evaluations assists in identifying interfering factors impacting the child's motor development, including social, emotional, behavioral, and/or cognitive deficits.

INTERVENTION

Occupational and Physical Therapy Services

Therapy services can be provided through the use of three models including direct, monitoring, or consultation (American Occupational Therapy Association [AOTA], 1987, 1989; Dunn & Campbell, 1991) in collaboration with a multidisciplinary, interdisciplinary, or transdisciplinary team approach. Direct intervention is assessment and intervention on a one-to-one basis between the therapist and child or a small group. In the monitoring service model, the therapist evaluates the child, develops a program, teaches an appropriate individual to carry out that program, and is directly responsible for monitoring the success/outcome of the therapy program (Dunn & Campbell, 1991). Consultation consists of the therapist consulting/sharing expertise directly with a teacher about a particular child or providing useful information to facilities (medical, educational, residential, etc.) through formal presentation to improve services in general. In this service model, the person/facility receiving the consultation is responsible for the outcome of the program (Dunn & Campbell, 1991). The therapist typically employs a combination of these therapy models to ensure the best outcome for a child and family.

Current federal legislation impacts the way occupational and physical therapy services are provided. Public Law 94-142 (1975), the Education of the Handicapped Act (EHA), addresses school-age children. This law mandates free and appropriate public education, as well as therapy services, if these related services are deemed necessary for a child to benefit from special education programming. Therapy services are detailed in the individualized education program (IEP).

Public Law 99-457 (1986), an amendment to the EHA, addresses infants and toddlers under Part H and preschoolers under Part B. Under Part H the parents are an integral part of the intervention process, and an individualized family service plan (IFSP) is designed by an interdisciplinary team and the parents. Occupational and physical therapy services are considered primary early intervention services, and therapy goals documented in the IFSP address needs of both child and family. Part H programs are currently discretionary for each state; federal funds are provided as incentives for development of appropriate early intervention programs. Under Part B, federal monies are available to states providing special education and related services, including occupational and physical therapy, for preschool children ages 3 through 5 years. Services are made available to preschoolers with identified disabilities.

CONCLUSION

This chapter provided an overview of typical and atypical motor development. Consistent with the neurodevelopmental principles outlined in Chapter 1, we have underscored that children with delays in motor development manifest primary neurologically based disabling conditions. We have described motor function as controlled by three major areas of the brain, including the cerebral cortex and upper motor neuron, cerebellum, and basal ganglia, and have described the particular dysfunctional implications of each. This might leave the impression that motor dysfunction is manifest in discrete observable patterns. Motor dysfunction is more typically mixed, meaning that complex patterns of dysfunction will be observed in the same child. Mixtures of hypo- and hypertonus can be observed between various parts of the body (for example truncal hypotonus with peripheral hypertonus) and will occur simultaneously with dyscoordination of movement and postural abnormalities.

Other primary neurologically based disabling conditions will occur in combination with these mixed motor deficits. The chief considerations in this regard are cognitive and speech/language dysfunction. As discussed in chapters 3 and 4, cognitive and speech/language dysfunction will similarly be "mixed." As a result, it is necessary to decide to what extent inability to perform a task stems from motor as opposed to cognitive dysfunction (dissociation). Finally, as will be discussed in Chapters 5 and 6, motor dysfunction, with or without associated cognitive and speech/language dysfunction, has important ramifications for behavioral, emotional, and family wellness.

CHAPTER 3

CHILDREN WITH COGNITIVE IMPAIRMENT

Stephen R. Hooper, Ph.D.
Kimberlee Berry-Sawyer, Ph.D.
Janice Howard, Ph.D.
Frederick List, Ph.D.
George W. Hynd, Ph.D.

From the preceding chapters it should be clear that children exhibiting developmental delay typically show multiple areas of primary neurological involvement. Even when there is a well defined neurological deficit, as seen in a child with motor involvement, a multitude of other problems can arise secondary to that specific deficit (e.g., low self-esteem, reluctance to engage in selected academic tasks). This supposition also holds for children showing primary cognitive impairment. Children with wide-ranging levels and patterns of cognitive functioning will show associated deficits and, importantly, *associated strengths*. Identifying the level of functioning and recognizing the associated pattern of strengths and weaknesses are crucial to gaining an increased understanding of how a child is functioning. This information also is

paramount in developing treatment strategies. Many other issues discussed in Chapter 1 clearly arise in children with cognitive impairment
(e.g., primary disabling conditions can be accompanied by secondary
social-emotional manifestations). For most of these children, the interdisciplinary approach is crucial to working in an effective manner with
these children.

This chapter provides an overview of the child with cognitive
impairment. The chapter begins with a discussion of several models that
have been purported to explain cognitive functioning. If one believes
that cognitive impairment is neurologically based, then it becomes important to know how various theorists conceptualize cognitive functioning. The following section addresses factors that can affect cognitive
functioning. Endogenous (e.g., sensory impairment, mental status) as
well as exogenous (e.g., environment) factors will be discussed. Most
of this chapter is devoted to describing, from a cognitive perspective,
several key neurodevelopmental disorders that confront clinicians and
researchers: mental retardation, pervasive developmental disorders,
learning disabilities, and attention-deficit hyperactivity disorder (ADHD).
This chapter concludes with a brief discussion of specific assessment
strategies and related clinical issues, in addition to a number of "rules
of thumb."

COMPONENTS OF COGNITION

Before describing the various kinds of cognitive impairment that individuals can manifest, it is important to understand the various hypothesized components of cognition. Cognition is multidimensional and goes
beyond any single measure depicting it, such as is typically expressed
by IQ scores. Although there is value in obtaining an overall level of
functioning (i.e., IQ), it is not reasonable nor helpful to reduce the many
facets of cognition into a single number. Factor analyses of many different types of testing batteries have yielded multidimensional solutions
(e.g., Sutter, Bishop, & Batten, 1986).

As such, several key theoretical models of cognition are presented,
each with its own unique conceptualization of cognition. Although these
descriptions are not intended to be exhaustive, the material provides an
overview of the multidimensionality of cognition.

Guilford's Structure of Intellect

Cognitive theorists have used various models to attempt to define and
explain human intelligence. Historically, one group of investigators

employed factor analysis to develop theories of intelligence, although these investigators generally were divided into those who believed in a general factor theory (i.e., g factor; Spearman, 1927), those who believed that intelligence was multifactorial (Horn, 1985; Thorndike, 1927), and those who believed in a combination (Thurstone, 1938; Vernon, 1950).

Perhaps the most cited model was proposed by J. P. Guilford (1967). Guilford was a prominent multifactor theorist who developed a three-dimensional model of the structure of intellect (SOI). One dimension represented the operations used for processing information. A second dimension represented the contents being processed, and a third dimension represented the products as the result of processing.

In addition, Guilford defined five different operations employed in his structure of intellect model. These included cognition (i.e., immediate awareness of information), memory, divergent production (i.e., creativity), convergent production (i.e., analytical thinking), and evaluation. Four types of content also were defined that included figural, symbolic, semantic, and behavioral (e.g., social cues). Finally, there were six types of products, consisting of units, classes, relations, systems, transformations, and implications.

This model produced a possible 120 cognitive factors: five types of operations × four types of contents × six types of products. The type of mental operation performed on a type of content yielded a resulting product. An example would be cognition (operation) of semantic (content) units (products). There is no general factor of intelligence in Guilford's SOI model. Guilford and his associates used factor analytic methods on performance tests to prove the existence of many, but not all of the factors that he defined. In addition, this model has been applied to many traditional intelligence tests, such as the *Wechsler Intelligence Scales for Children* and the *Wechsler Preschool and Primary Scales of Intelligence.*

Luria's Neuropsychological Model

Cognitive psychology, neuropsychology, and related disciplines have presented a variety of terms for a dichotomous information processing model. These terms have included successive versus simultaneous (Das, Kirby, & Jarman, 1979; Luria, 1966), analytic versus holistic (Bogen, 1969), sequential versus synchronous (Pavio, 1976), controlled versus automatic (Schneider & Shiffrin, 1977), and time ordered versus time dependent (Gordon & Bogen, 1974). Two information processing styles are presented which take the emphasis off content and place it on the information processing itself (Kaufman, 1979).

Luria (1970) proposed a functional model of brain organization that has been embraced by many professionals. Luria (1966) was one of the first investigators to advance a dichotomous view of information processing. Based on neuropsychological data, much support has been generated regarding the successive versus simultaneous processing aspects of this model (Das et al., 1979).

Simultaneous information processing has been described as involving stimuli having spatial components. It refers to the synthesis of separate elements into groups. The fundamental nature of this type of processing is that any portion of the result is at once surveyable without dependence on its position in the whole (Das et al., 1979). Simultaneous processing is necessary to form any holistic gestalt and has been associated with many tasks that demand spatial and/or visuoconstructive abilities. Luria (1966) categorized simultaneous processing into three types. The first type is *direct perception*. The process of perception is such that the individual is selectively attentive to the stimulus input in the brain. Accordingly, this type of information is primarily spatial. The second type, *mnestic processes*, refers to the organization of stimulus traces from earlier experiences. These traces can be either short-term or long term and the integration of the traces occurs on the basis of criteria internal or external to the individual. The third type is found in *complex intellectual processes*. Thus, for the individual to comprehend systems of relationships, it is necessary that the components of the system be represented simultaneously (Das et al., 1979).

Successive information processing involves the integration of stimuli into some temporally organized arrangement. Each stimulus is related in a linear fashion to the preceding and following ones. Important here is the notion that a stimulus is not totally surveyable at any one point. With this type of processing, a system of cues consecutively activates the components of the whole (Das et al., 1979). As with simultaneous processing, successive processing has perceptual, mnestic, and complex intellectual components. Tasks most frequently used to tap successive processing include serial recall of words and numbers.

Luria (1966) and others (e.g., Das et al., 1979) considered the successive or sequential type of processing to be a function of the frontotemporal regions of the brain and the simultaneous processing to be mediated by the occipitoparietal regions. This thinking is in contrast to that of Bogen (1969), Gazzaniga (1975), and Nebes (1975) who associate the sequential types of processing with the left cerebral hemisphere and simultaneous processing with the right hemisphere.

On the localization of these information processing strategies, it is important to note that Luria (1966) stated that simultaneous and successive processing could not be totally identified with specific modalities (e.g., visual, auditory, tactile perception). The processing in these components is not necessarily affected by sensory input. Visual information can be processed successively and auditory information can be processed simultaneously. Both types of information processing, however, can be involved in all forms of responding. Further, it has been suggested that there is probably an interplay between the two processing systems (Das et al., 1979).

The simultaneous versus successive information processing model has yielded meaningful evidence on information processing strategies of normal children (Kirby & Das, 1977), children with mild (Blackman, Bilsky, Burger, & Mar, 1976; Cummins & Das, 1980) and moderate (Klanderman & Kaplan, 1982) mental retardation, and children with learning disabilities (Das, Leong, & Williams, 1978). Cummins and Das (1977) have proposed a framework for research on developmental disabilities using this information processing model.

Gardner's Model

A recent theory of intelligence that has gained popular support was proposed more than 10 years ago by Gardner (1983). His theory challenged the dichotomous structure of intelligence (simultaneous versus successive; verbal versus nonverbal abilities). Rather than deriving a theory based on statistical manipulation of data sets, Gardner proposed a theory that was based on neuropsychological evidence on the manner in which the human brain and nervous system function.

Gardner does not believe that there is sufficient evidence to support the view of a central executive system that directs all mental activity. According to Gardner, the available evidence gained from neuropsychological data suggests the existence of multiple intellectual capabilities. Although they do interact in various ways to produce a wide array of observable human talents, each is believed to be relatively autonomous.

Gardner has proposed the existence of seven distinct intellectual capabilities. He allows for the possibility of more to be discovered. Of the seven, the first two are those that are typically assessed in traditional intellectual evaluations: *linguistic* intelligence, which includes the understanding of semantics, a sensitivity to phonology, and a knowledge of syntax, and *logical-mathematical* intelligence. This latter type of intelligence is responsible for an individual's ability to perform numerical calculations and to grasp the logic within mathematical formulas.

Traditionally, three of the proposed capabilities have been viewed as talents rather than as forms of intelligence. *Musical* intelligence is reflected in the ability to master rhythm and pitch. It is expressed through musical composition as well as vocal and instrumental performance. Gardner (1983) stated that, "Of all the gifts with which individuals may be endowed, none emerges earlier than musical talent" (p. 99). Another form of intelligence that Gardner proposed is *spatial*. This includes the abilities for accurately perceiving the visual world, performing transformations and/or modifications on the initial perception, and recreating some part of that visual experience, even when the relevant physical stimuli are not present. *Bodily-kinesthetic* is another proposed form of intelligence that others have often considered as a type of talent. This form of intelligence is related to many human physical activities including dancing, athletics, mime, and the work of inventors. All of these forms share the common "ability to use one's body in highly differentiated and skilled ways, for expressive as well as goal-directed purposes" (Gardner, 1983, p. 206).

Gardner's final two types of intelligence are, perhaps, the ones that are most different from those abilities that are typically associated with intelligence. Together they are known as the personal intelligences. *Intrapersonal* intelligence is an awareness of one's own emotions. It includes an understanding of one's range of emotions, the ability to discriminate between emotions and to label them, and the capability to use the emotions to help in understanding and directing one's behavior. *Interpersonal* intelligence is the outward focusing of similar abilities. It includes the ability to differentiate individuals particularly based on their moods, temperaments, motivations, and intentions.

Although Gardner's theory has been viewed as a distinct departure from the more traditional models of intelligence, it appears to incorporate the traditional concept of stability. He does not address this issue directly, but it does appear that the proposed intelligences have a strong biological basis that remains relatively constant over the course of one's life (Feldman & Adams, 1989). If the proposed intelligences display a high degree of stability, then it should be possible to assess them during the early stages of development and predict, with a high degree of accuracy, the relative strength of each intelligence over time, using the same approaches as with the more traditional psychometric assessments.

Although explicit evaluation procedures have not yet been designed to assess each of the individual intelligences, Gardner believes that a child's individual intellectual abilities may be assessed best through planned observations. For example, observations of a child performing a set of selected age-appropriate tasks could be conducted for 5–10 hours over the course of a month. Gardner believes that these observational procedures could be used to develop a profile of a child's areas of strengths and weaknesses. This profile could be used to help in planning the child's educational needs.

Sternberg's Triarchic Model

Sternberg's triarchic theory of intelligence (Sternberg, 1988) can be classified under the information processing models that focus on ways in which individuals process and store information. Sternberg's theory attempts to explain specific information processes that operate in given contexts, and presents intelligence as a rough estimate of an individual's ability to process information at a given point in time (Feldman & Adams, 1989). Thus, intelligence is something that is malleable, not fixed, and can be improved over time.

Sternberg (1986) defined intelligence as the "purposive adaptation to, selection of, and shaping of real-world environments relevant to one's life and abilities." Therefore, the triarchic theory is so named because it attempts to deal with intelligence in its relationship with three main areas of an individual's life: *Componential* (i.e., the relationship between intelligence and the internal world of the individual); *Experiential* (i.e., the relationship between intelligence and the experience of the individual); and *Contextual* (i.e., the relationship between intelligence and the external world of the individual). Further, the triarchic theory describes the relationship of intelligence to the internal world of the individual, (i.e., the mental mechanisms involved in thinking), as composed of three basic kinds of information processing: metacomponents, performance components, and knowledge-acquisition components. These three processes are interdependent and work in an integrative fashion.

Metacomponents are considered by Sternberg to be "white collar" components, being the higher-order, executive processes used to plan what one is doing, monitor action, and evaluate the action on completion (Sternberg, 1988). Specific metacomponents are limited in number and include (1) recognizing the existence of a problem, (2) deciding the nature of the problem, (3) selecting a set of lower-order processes to solve the problem, (4) selecting a strategy into which to combine these components, (5) selecting a mental representation on which the components and strategy can act, (6) allocating one's mental resources, (7) monitoring one's problem solving as it is happening, and (8) evaluating one's problem solving after it is done (Sternberg, 1988).

Performance components are considered the "blue collar" information processing components (Sternberg, 1988) in that the elements execute instructions of the metacomponents. Unlike metacomponents, the number of performance components is quite large, with each component specific to narrow ranges of tasks. Essentially, the performance components actively solve problems according to the plans commanded by the metacomponents. Examples of performance components include encoding, inference, mapping, application, justification, and response in the inductive reasoning modality.

Knowledge-acquisition components are "the students of mental self-management" (Sternberg, 1988) and are used to learn new information. Eventually, the metacomponents and performance components will automatically perform this newly acquired information for a non-novel situation, thus making an individual more mentally effective. Specific knowledge-acquisition components include selective encoding, selective combination, and selective comparison (Sternberg, 1988).

According to the triarchic theory, the relationship between intelligence and experience (experiential) is equally important in understanding one's intelligence. Within this domain, assessing intelligence requires one to consider not only the information processing components involved (e.g., metacomponents, performance components, knowledge-acquisition components), but the experience to which they are applied. The ability to cope with relative novelty and to automatize newly acquired information are considered essential aspects of intelligence in how individuals successfully relate to their environments.

Intelligence, as it relates to an individual's external world (contextual), is intelligent thought directed toward the goals of adaptation to one's existing environment, the shaping of one's environment, and to the selection of one's environment (Sternberg, 1988). Essentially, most intelligent thought is purposeful and is directed toward an individual's attempt to adapt to one's environment. This adaptation can vary and should be evaluated according to an individual's culture.

Essentially, the triarchic theory of intelligence asserts that the different components account for overall intellectual development. Specifically, the metacomponents activate the performance and knowledge acquisition components that, in turn, provide feedback to the metacomponents. In addition, the knowledge-acquisition components increase an individual's adaptation to, selection of, and shaping of one's environment. Finally, with the application of these components to new experiences, fewer tasks remain novel, allowing more time and attention for dealing with novel tasks and situations. Therefore, an individual adapts and becomes a more effective mental manager of their environment (Sternberg, 1988).

The triarchic theory lends itself to serving predictive and diagnostic functions. The recently proposed *Sternberg Triarchic Abilities Test* (1988) serves to assess each ability delineated by the triarchic theory (excepting environmental shaping and selection functions of the contextual aspect). This set of procedures provides information about a subject's specific skills and abilities, as well as information regarding the strengths and weaknesses of the individual. These types of information help an individual deal more effectively within any selected environment.

Summary

As can be seen from the preceding discussion, there is no clear universally accepted conceptualization of cognition. Each of the models detailed illustrates the multidimensionality of cognitive process. None of the models presents simplistic conceptualizations typically used in traditional tests of intelligence (e.g., the *Wechsler Intelligence Scale for Children-III* provides a verbal IQ, performance, IQ, and a full scale IQ). It also should be clear that within each model, each component is linked to one another in unknown ways, thus supporting the notion that a problem in one component may lead to problems in other components. Further, given a neurological insult or maldevelopment, the functioning and/or developmental trajectory of these components can be altered in yet unpredictable ways. Consequently, the assessment and tracking of these functions are important aspects in working with children with cognitive impairments. Professionals who work with individuals with developmental disabilities should be aware of the multidimensional nature of intelligence and sensitive to the many different profiles that can be manifested.

FACTORS AFFECTING COGNITIVE FUNCTION

There are a variety of factors that can affect the integrity and/or efficiency of an individual's cognitive function. It is essential that professionals rule out sensory impairments before determining a child's cognitive function. Professionals should be particularly attentive to the possibility of intercurrent sensory impairments in settings of significant developmental delay. In such settings, sensory impairments are easily overlooked.

Another factor that can drastically influence a child's cognitive functioning is the presence of emotional disturbance. Whether primary or secondary in nature or neurologic and/or psychiatric in origin, clearly emotional problems can interfere with cognitive efficiency, motor speed, and general attention to task. Further, a child's strengths may be lessened by emotional disturbance and any cognitive weaknesses may be worsened. Rourke (1989) has proposed a neurologically based model that incorporates a selected pattern of neuropsychological dysfunction, affective disruption, and academic deficits. This model identified right hemisphere-based neuropsychological deficits, depressive symptoms, and specific deficits in arithmetic. Although this model continues to be examined with respect to efficacy, it remains that children with cognitive dysfunction will manifest a wide array of emotional problems. These problems can have a negative affect on the assessment of cognitive function.

The environment also can affect a child's cognitive functioning. Professionals working with children having developmental disabilities should be sure to gain information about such areas of the child's home environment as educational values, literacy, family stability, and financial resources. This information is helpful in determining if environmental deprivation or neglect has affected a child's cognitive development. Relatedly, professionals should be careful when evaluating children who lack exposure to a culture's primary language. For example, in homes where English is the second language, modifications in assessment strategies should be used (e.g., involving the primary caregiver in the assessment process).

COGNITIVELY BASED DISORDERS

Mental Retardation: Identification Issues

Mental retardation is a descriptive term implying that a child so affected shows significant deviation from the course of normal mental and social-adaptive development. In Chapter 1 we described the Gesell framework of developmental dysfunction, encompassing motor skills, visual perception/problem solving, language, and social/adaptive behavior. Using this framework, the generalist conceptualizes cognitive functioning as representing a combination of visual perception/problem solving and language, and conceptualizes social-adaptive behavior as the manifestation of the combination of visual perception/problem solving, language, *and* motor skills. Mental retardation, therefore, becomes the prototype of cognitive disorders in the sense that the most common pattern of disorder is anticipated to be that in which there occurs coordinated deficits of both visual perception/problem-solving and language skills. Mild degrees of dysfunction are expected to predominate over more severe degrees. Appreciation of these developmental distinctions is important as we look at some contemporary definitions of mental retardation.

The American Association of Mental Retardation has defined mental retardation in terms of low intelligence (i.e., overall intelligence scores at least two standard deviations below the mean on an individually administered intelligence test), deficits in adaptive behavior, and onset of retardation occurring before the eighteenth birthday (Grossman, 1983). This basic definition was adopted by the current version of the *Diagnostic and Statistical Manual of Mental Disorders, DSM-III-R,* (American Psychiatric Association, 1987). The *DSM-III-R* also defines four degrees of severity based on the level of intellectual functioning: Mild: IQ = 50–70; Moderate: IQ = 35–50; Severe: IQ = 20–35; Profound: IQ <20.

The American Association of Mental Retardation has adopted a new definition of mental retardation that emphasizes the degree of support that an individual requires and deemphasizes the focus on IQ, seen in previous definitions (Turkington, 1993). According to this new definition, subaverage intellectual function must exist concurrently with related limitations in two or more of the following applicable adaptive skill areas: communication, self-care, home living, social skills, community use, self-direction, health and safety, functional academics, leisure, and work. Mental retardation also must manifest before age 18 (Turkington, 1993). Additionally, rather than defining the degree of severity based on intellectual level, the new definition defines four intensity levels of required support: intermittent, limited, extensive, and pervasive.

From the perspective of the generalist, it is expected that children with cognitive deficits will exhibit similar problems in the two major domains related to cognitive function, namely visual perception/problem solving and language. When the generalist considers definitions of mental retardation related to adaptive function, it should be appreciated that this is a combination of motor and cognitive domains. It should be obvious how these issues relate to the information gathered from the neurodevelopmental history and examination in clarifying the relative impact of cognition and motor related to "mental retardation."

Cognitive Models of Mental Retardation

Ellis (1970) proposed a model of memory and cognitive functioning that has been used in studying areas of deficits related to mental retardation. Ellis proposed four stages of memory that differ in the amount of time information is retained in the storage capacity. The first stage is called very short-term memory (VSTM), which is the sensory representation of stimuli. Information is maintained in this stage for a very brief period. Primary memory (PM) is often referred to as short-term memory. It has a limited capacity and maintains information for a slightly longer period of time than the VSTM. Secondary memory (SM) can hold more information for a longer period than PM. Various rehearsal strategies are used to transfer information to and from SM. Tertiary memory (TM) is described as the long-term storage of over-learned information. Its capacity is limitless, as is its duration. A person may be unable to retrieve information, however, because of difficulties in the use of retrieval strategies or some nature of interference. Ellis also proposed two processes that are responsible for the movement of information between memory stages. Attentional/perceptual processes are used to transfer the information from VSTM to PM. The rehearsal processes, as previously noted, are important for recirculating information through PM to maintain it. These strategies also are used to move information from PM to SM.

Research has suggested that individuals with mental retardation perform much more poorly than nonretarded individuals on tasks measuring short-term sensory and perceptual processing (Borkowski, Peck, & Damberg, 1983). When faced with a task requiring them to discriminate between two objects based on a specific physical characteristic, individuals with mental retardation appear to require more time to accumulate a sufficient amount of sensory information to make a correct discrimination (Lally & Nettlebeck, 1977). However, evidence does not support the presence of structural deficits in the VSTM. On the contrary, the ability of individuals with mental retardation to perceive stimuli in their environment appears equivalent to that of nonretarded individuals. The studies that have shown differences in this area have related their findings to perceptual processing difficulties, as previously noted, as well as deficits in attention (Stanovich, 1978).

Although there is general agreement that individuals with mental retardation typically manifest attentional deficits, it is unclear what aspect of cognitive processing is affected by these deficits. Nettlebeck and Brewer (1981) conclude that inferior performance of individuals with mental retardation on a reaction time task resulted from a general attention deficit that affected all aspects of information processing from creating a state of preparedness to encoding the perceptual stimulus, translating the stimulus into memory, and finally processing the appropriate response. Others have shown that the attention deficit has more limited effects, primarily related to a less efficient conscious allocation or maintenance of attention to pertinent stimuli (Borkowski et al., 1983; Hagan & Huntsman, 1971; Merril, 1992; Zeaman & House, 1979). Tomporowski, Hayden, and Applegate (1990) found that subjects with mental retardation demonstrated an ability to sustain their attention equivalent to that of nonretarded subjects, although the subjects with dysfunction were more likely to commit more errors of omission and commission. These findings are consistent with other findings regarding an inefficient use of attention.

Primary memory abilities also have been investigated. Ellis (1970) concluded that there was no difference between subjects with and without mental retardation, based on equal performances in recalling the last items from a list of test items (i.e., recency effect). Zeaman and House (1979), however, indicated that the capacity of the short-term memory was negatively related to the level of intelligence. Tomporowski et al. (1990) also found a deficit in the short-term memory of individuals with mental retardation when they were engaged in a task requiring sustained attention.

Most studies that have investigated SM have focused on the degree to which individuals with mental retardation can use rehearsal strategies in an efficient manner. Although Ellis (1970) failed to find a difference in the recency effect, his results did reveal a significant difference in the primacy effect (i.e., memory of the initial items on a list of stimulus words). He believed that this reflected SM deficits in individuals with mental retardation. He also examined the effect of increased exposure time to the stimulus words on recall in subjects with mental retardation. He found that there was no improvement in recall. He concluded that the subjects failed to use active rehearsal. This failure to spontaneously use active rehearsal strategies to memorize information more effectively also has been observed in other studies (Brown, 1974; Davies, Sperber, & McCauley, 1981). There are some mental activities, however, that do not require a significant degree of conscious, active processing. Such activities are typically overlearned behaviors that can be accomplished through a more automatic process (e.g., reading letters, tying shoes). Although automatic processing does not appear to be related to the level of intellectual functioning, evidence indicates that individuals with mental retardation may require more time to learn basic tasks to the point of becoming automatic (Sperber & McCauley, 1984). A study that has examined one type of automatic processing focused on spatial memory (Ellis, Woodley-Zanthos, & Dulaney, 1989). The results of that study supported the belief that there are no differences in passive processing related to level of intellectual functioning.

Some studies have attempted to explore relationships between intelligence and TM. Most studies, however, appear to have too many methodologic problems, preventing making sound conclusions about differences in TM related to intellectual level (Detterman, 1979). Because of all of the claims regarding the presence of deficits in earlier stages of the memory process, it even has been questioned if TM could be measured accurately (Borkowski et al., 1983).

Because of the various cognitive deficits that have been found in individuals with mental retardation, interest has developed in exploring the degree to which the deficits could be overcome. Some studies have found that the deficits could be reduced by explicit instructions in cognitive strategies, although the extent of the improvement has been limited (Borkowski et al., 1983). The areas most often focused on have been the abilities to maintain the strategies learned and to transfer the strategies to different tasks. Results of studies have varied, depending on the type of task in which the individuals were trained. Baroody (1988) found that subjects with moderate mental retardation displayed a good ability to retain and transfer their training in rule-based number comparison. This training focused on improving their ability to gauge the relative magnitude of two numbers. Other studies have found that, although training can have some short-term benefit, it can be difficult to attain long-term maintenance.

There is even less likelihood that an individual with mental retardation can transfer the newly acquired skill independently to tasks that are different from the one used in the training (Campione, Brown, Ferrara, Jones, & Steinberg, 1985; Day & Hall, 1988). Some training has been found to result in a degree of cognitive rigidity or inertia. Some studies attempted to determine if individuals with mental retardation could be trained to develop an automated response on a visual interference task (Ellis & Dulaney, 1991; Ellis, Woodley-Zanthos, Dulaney, & Palmer, 1989). The subjects demonstrated an ability equal to that of nonretarded individuals in developing the automated response; however, they had greater difficulty with persisting in the trained response style even when the nature of the task was changed such that the trained response was no longer beneficial. The effects of the cognitive inertia were found to persist for more than 3 months in most of the subjects with mental retardation, yet it disappeared in less than a month for the nonretarded subjects. Consequently, although it appears possible to help individuals with mental retardation overcome some of their cognitive deficits, it is necessary to use training that is task-specific, provide an ample of amount of training to assist in mastery of the task, and be prepared to assist the individual in learning to apply the training to different tasks or to make necessary changes when the nature of the task changes.

Communication Disorders

The child with a communication disorder manifests a delay in connected language understanding and usage. Language dysfunction can occur in settings in which there is diffuse cognitive dysfunction, meaning that the disability in language is accompanied by a corresponding degree of perceptual dysfunction, and in settings in which the cognitive deficit appears to occur primarily in language. When language dysfunction is accompanied by a corresponding degree of visual perceptual dysfunction we refer to the language disability as occurring within a setting of mental retardation. Here there is no disproportionate disability in language and the child may appear significantly slow in cognitive skills, including language. When there occurs a disproportionate delay in language development compared with visual perceptual development, one begins to encounter certain oddities or peculiarities of behavior. Behavioral variations noted in children with disproportionate delays in language function relative to visual perceptual function include:

1. *Inconsistent eye contact.* When confronted verbally, the child typically exhibits only brief eye contact. The child may look about the room fixing only briefly on visual objects of interest.
2. *Differential in auditory and visual attention span.* The child with discrepant language dysfunction may tend to ignore auditory stimuli, especially when visually occupied. The child will behave as if having a hearing problem, but audiologic assessment will convey normal hearing with a failure to attend to auditory stimuli.
3. *Perseveration on visual problem-solving items.* The child will exhibit inordinate fascination and fixation on tasks involving manipulation of objects. For example, the child may make involved and intricate designs with blocks or by drawing, may show inordinate attention to visual detail and so on.
4. *Frustration when confronted verbally.* The child with discrepant language dysfunction will exhibit increasing frustration when confronted verbally and may tend to avoid confrontational language situations.

What is obvious from this list of behaviors observed in children with discrepant language function (compared with visual perceptual abilities) is that many of these same behaviors are observed in children with infantile autism.

Autistic Disorder

Leo Kanner (1943) originally described the autistic syndrome as including an inability to relate to people in ordinary ways, superior rote memory skills, under- or overdeveloped sensitivity to noise, perseverative behavior and desire for sameness in routine, lack of spontaneous activity, and normal cognitive potential. Approximately 50% of children with autism never develop functional speech (Rutter, 1965) and those with speech may exhibit one or more of the following characteristics: invariation in tone or pitch of voice, mechanical-sounding utterances, sing-song voice quality, repeating previously heard stereotyped phrases, lack of reciprocal conversation with others, and conversation limited in depth and range of interests. Other behavioral manifestations include lack of eye contact and/or coordinated eye gaze with vocalizations, lack of pretend or imaginary play, lack of awareness of others' feelings, restricted range of interests in activities, sensory interests (i.e., visual, auditory, tactile, smell, and taste), difficulty modulating sensory information, and stereotypic body movements (e.g., rocking, hand mannerisms).

In general, all autistic children will be communicatively disordered in that connected language understanding will be disproportionately delayed compared with other aspects of cognitive development. Similarly, all communicatively disordered children will have some autistic-like behaviors. However, not all communicatively disordered children will have enough autistic-like behaviors (i.e., be far enough along the autistic number line or rating scale) to be labeled "autistic." Nonetheless, the essence of being autistic is to be communicatively disordered.

The incidence of autistic disorder is approximately 4 to 10 in 10,000 (Gillberg & Gillberg, 1989). The incidence of mental retardation is approximately 3 in 100. This suggests that autistic disorder is significantly (approximately 100 times) less common than mental retardation.

Learning Disabilities

Learning disabilities are primary neurologically based handicapping conditions with a significant discrepancy between cognitive abilities and academic achievement. Kirk (1963) is originally credited with coining of the term "learning disability." However, the conceptualization of childhood learning disorders has spanned nearly 100 years, dating back to Morgan's (1896) case of "congenital word blindness." It was not until 1975 that the 94th U.S. Congress put forth the first widely accepted definition of learning disabilities. This definition stated that the learning disabled child experiences:

> a disorder in one or more of the basic psychological processes involved in understanding or in using language, spoken or written, which may manifest itself in an imperfect ability to listen, think, speak, read, write, spell, or do mathematical

calculation. The term includes such conditions as perceptual handicaps, brain injury, minimal brain dysfunction, dyslexia, and developmental aphasia. (U.S. Office of Education, 1976, p. 56977)

This definition was adopted by most state education departments and, being a legal mandate, carried with it numerous due process procedures and regulations. Although not fully detailed, this definition did allude to the involvement of some form of neurological dysfunction in the child with learning disability. This definition was important in setting the tone for the study of learning disabilities, but it remained sufficiently general in its description that the definition has since been considered inadequate.

The most recent definition of learning disabilities was proposed over 6 years ago by the Interagency Committee on Learning Disabilities (ICLD) (1987), a multidisciplinary group mandated by the Health Research Extension Act of 1985 (P.L. 99-158). This definition stated that:

Learning disabilities is a generic term that refers to a heterogeneous group of disorders manifested by significant difficulties in the acquisition and use of listening, speaking, reading, writing, reasoning, or mathematical abilities, or of social skills. These disorders are intrinsic to the individual and presumed to be due to central nervous system dysfunction. Even though a learning disability may occur concomitantly with other handicapping conditions (e.g., sensory impairment, mental retardation, social and emotional disturbance), with socioenvironmental influences (e.g., cultural differences, insufficient or inappropriate instruction, psychogenic factors), and especially with attention deficit disorder, all of which may cause learning problems, a learning disability is not the direct result of those conditions or influences. (ICLD, 1987, p. 222)

Although this definition includes the core components of its predecessor, it also presents additional conceptual and practical concerns for the generalist. Specifically, this definition includes deficiencies in social skills within the parameters of learning disabilities. Similarly, the inclusion of sociocultural influences in the definition, along with the impact of ADHD also provide for additional diagnostic dilemmas for those working with individuals with learning problems. The U.S. Department of Education has not endorsed the ICLD definition given the many concerns and issues raised by this proposed definition.

Although the conceptualization of learning disabilities has progressed from attempts to identify a single underlying cause (e.g., pathological cerebral dominance, specific perceptual deficits) to attempts to implicate multiple, perhaps interactive, factors, the issue of obtaining a reliable subtyping scheme remains a major obstacle today. Nonetheless, the research has progressed to the point of delineating between different types of learning problems. Although this research has been reviewed extensively elsewhere (e.g., Hooper & Willis, 1989; Feagan, Short, & Meltzer, 1991), a cursory review of these trends is in order.

Reading Subtypes

Within the reading domain, there is support for at least two different subtypes of reading difficulty (Bakker, 1973; Pirozzolo, 1979). The first subtype that is consistently described demonstrates auditory-linguistic deficits, but intact visual-spatial abilities. This group of deficient readers experiences primary deficits in letter-sound integration and poor use of phonetic word decoding strategies. Other linguistic deficits also may be found in this subtype pattern (e.g., poor semantics). This is the largest group of disabled readers (Boder, 1970; Mattis, French, & Rapin, 1975).

A second subtype that has been described manifests the opposite pattern of the auditory-linguistic group. In this subtype, auditory processing and linguistic abilities are intact, but visual-spatial difficulties are pronounced. These children have primary deficiencies in perceiving whole words as gestalts and may even over-phoneticize in their word decoding. This subtype is more rare than the auditory-linguistic subtype (Boder, 1970; Mattis et al., 1975), perhaps because of the emphasis on auditory and linguistic strategies in traditional classroom instruction.

Some investigators have insisted on a third diagnostic subtype, incorporating characteristics of the auditory-linguistic and visual-spatial subtypes (e.g., Bateman, 1968; Boder, 1970; Satz & Morris, 1981), although others have attempted to include motor and sensory deficits in their subtype models (Fisk & Rourke, 1979; Lyon & Watson, 1981; Mattis et al., 1975). Many different reading patterns likely exist, but their operational definitions remain elusive.

Spelling Subtypes

Research in this academic area has consistently yielded two subtypes of disabled spellers (Naidoo, 1972; Nelson & Warrington, 1974; Sweeney & Rourke, 1978). One of the subtypes exhibits reading and spelling deficiencies and suggests the possible presence of a more pervasive language disorder. Children in the second subtype have managed to overcome their initial reading problems, but they remain poor spellers. This subtype of deficient spellers has been described as not using lexical, or letter-by-letter processing in learning to spell, thus implicating phonological processing problems (Frith, 1983). Sweeney and Rourke

(1978) elucidated that poor spellers are more effectively discriminated from good spellers across many neuropsychological tasks, particularly at older age levels. Further, those spellers who evidenced the use of phonetic principles, even in their spelling errors, seem to have a better academic prognosis. Further validation of spelling subtypes, particularly as relating to prognosis and treatment strategies, is required.

Written Language Subtypes

Similar to the spelling subtypes, the area of written language has just begun to be examined with respect to its multidimensionality. Although many contemporary conceptual models have been advanced addressing the issue of written language subtypes (e.g., Abbott & Berninger, 1993; Ellis, 1982; Roeltgen, 1985), the conceptualization of writing as a multidimensional phenomenon dates to the mid-1800s (Ogle, 1867). Further, the evidence presented to date implicates a variety of neuro-psychological underpinnings influencing written language output. For example, Gregg (1992) notes that there are a variety of language-based processes (e.g., phonological disorders, dysnomia), visualspatial pro-cesses, and executive functions (e.g., organization, planning, evaluat-ing) that can affect written language functioning. Despite this rich history, however, there have been few studies demonstrating the multi-dimensional nature of written language.

Berninger, Mizokawa, and Bragg (1991) hypothesized that one kind of writing disability may involve the inability to translate knowledge or written language into an actual written product, despite the presence of intact functioning in other domains. A second kind of writing dis-ability is manifested by taking a long time to compose with few major inaccuracies in the actual output. Children manifesting this kind of defi-cit can be contrasted with those whose composing times may be inor-dinately slow and output is inaccurate. Two other kinds of writing difficulties can occur at the word level of analysis, with one kind show-ing a specific deficit in word production only and the other showing deficits in both word decision and word production. Specific treatment suggestions are put forth by Berninger et al. for each of these written language subtypes.

One of the first empirical studies to address the multidimensional nature of written expression in children and adolescents was conducted by Sandler et al. (1992). Based on teacher ratings of writing legibility, mechanics, writing rate, spelling, and written language sophistication, clinic-referred children, ages 9 to 15, were grouped into those having a writing disorder ($n = 99$) and those without ($n = 63$). All subjects received a neurodevelopmental battery designed to screen eight broad areas of functioning: minor neurologic indicators, fine motor function, language, gross motor function, temporal-sequential organization, visual processing, selective attention, and memory. Cluster analytic techniques produced six reliable clusters, four of which composed the writing disorder group.

The largest group (n = 50) evidenced fine-motor and linguistic deficits, with writing problems characterized by poor phonetic spelling, slow motor output, and problems with mechanics. The second group (n = 35) predominantly manifested visual-spatial deficits, with their writing being characterized by poor legibility and poor spatial organization. In contrast to the first group, however, children in the second group evidenced adequate spelling and idea generation. Group three (n = 9) showed prominent problems with attention and memory. Their writing was characterized by poor spelling with frequent omissions, insertions, and inconsistencies. Legibility, mechanics, and rate were generally intact. The final writing disorder group (n = 11) showed primary deficits in their sequencing and their written output was characterized by poor automatization of letter production, poor mechanics, and decreased legibility. Although this study could be criticized from many perspectives (e.g., sampling, assessment procedures), it is important in that it provides further support for the heterogeneous nature of written language dysfunction.

Arithmetic Subtypes

Subtypes of arithmetic disability also have begun to be examined. Over two decades ago Cohn (1971) stated that difficulties in mathematics could be attributable to a more pervasive language disorder. Rourke & Finlayson (1978), and Rourke & Strang (1978), have since provided evidence for subtypes of arithmetic disability. Using a wide range of instruments selected to tap the neuropsychological areas of tactile perception, visual perception, auditory perception, motor function, conceptual thinking, and academic achievement, Rourke and his colleagues described two statistically derived subtypes of arithmetic disability.

The first subtype provided support for Cohn's (1971) speculation that language deficits were primarily responsible for some difficulties in mathematics. This group manifested adequate understanding of basic arithmetic processes along with deficits in reading and/or spelling skills. These children exhibited neuropsychological deficits on verbally based tasks, but adequate visual-perceptual processing. Mathematical errors were characterized by inadequate comprehension of word problems and instructions, difficulties memorizing facts and step-by-step procedures, and inexperience with subject material, largely because of grade retentions and special education intervention focusing on other areas, such as reading. However, these children did seem to have an adequate understanding of basic arithmetic processes (Rourke & Strang, 1978).

The second subtype of arithmetic disabilities identified by Rourke and colleagues evidenced adequate reading and spelling skills. These children had adequately developed auditory-perceptual abilities, but deficient visual-perceptual, psychomotor, and tactile-perceptual abilities. In contrast to the first subtype, this arithmetic subtype had difficulties with the mechanical aspects of calculation, such as misreading procedural signs, misalignment of columns of numbers, neglection of numbers in the arithmetic process, and poor numerals formation. In addition, these children were poorly organized in performing arithmetical calculations, they did not check their work, and they did not always understand the arithmetic principle that they were using (Rourke & Strang, 1978).

Attention Deficit Disorders

We conceptualize ADHD as a primary neurologically based heterogeneous disabling condition toward the mild, diffuse end of the developmental disabilities spectrum. ADHD has been defined in the *DSM-III-R* as comprising developmentally inappropriate inattention, impulsivity, and hyperactivity, with an early onset in childhood (American Psychiatric Association, 1987). This disorder has received a great deal of attention in recent years, although there is considerable controversy on whether this disorder is a separate clinical entity.

Previously, we have talked about the broad aspects of motor and cognitive dysfunction in children. We have suggested that the most commonly observed patterns of developmental delay is that in which there occurs diffuse delay across motor, cognitive, and social-adaptive development and in which the delay across these multiple developmental domains is of mild as opposed to severe extent. Historically, these combined concepts of associated deficits of mild extent were incorporated in the concept of "minimal brain dysfunction" expounded in the early 1970s (Wender, 1971). The concept of minimal brain dysfunction acknowledged the presence of multiple subtle areas of neurological dysfunction in children; however, the term minimal brain dysfunction (as opposed to the concept) was very unpopular. It is unfortunate that ADHD, as defined in the *DSM-III-R*, focuses entirely on issues of attention and impulsivity and ignores associated, primary neurologically based deficits such as gross and fine motor dyscoordination (clumsiness), oral motor dyscoordination (misarticulation), and learning disabilities. It would be difficult to adequately conceptualize ADHD as a pure entity as described in the *DSM-III-R* without attending to these associated primary, neurologically based deficits.

Additionally, secondary behavioral and emotional problems typically co-occur in children with ADHD, and these include low self-esteem, mood lability, significant problems in social relations, low frustration tolerance, and temper outbursts (Guevremont & Barkley, 1992). In most cases, the course of this disorder persists throughout childhood and approximately one-third of children with ADHD show signs of the disorder in adulthood (Gittelman, Mannuzza, Shenker, & Bonagura, 1985). It is estimated that 25% of adults with ADHD have some form of antisocial personality disorder.

The incidence rates of ADHD in the general population range from 3% to 5% (American Psychiatric Association, 1987). Additionally, it has been estimated that approximately 30% to 40% of children referred to child mental health clinics present with ADHD symptomatology (Barkley, 1982) and represent one of the most common referral complaints to child mental health professionals in the United States (Ross & Ross, 1982). Sex ratios indicate that 5 to 10 times as many males are diagnosed with these problems when compared to females (Holborrow, Berry, & Elkins, 1984), although one must consider that the criteria of ADHD may not exclude developmentally normal male behaviors at younger ages (Pennington, 1991).

There are many theories and predisposing factors that have attempted to explain the cause or causes of ADHD; however, at present, there is no single known etiology that accounts for the wide range of symptom manifestation in ADHD (Guevremont & Barkley, 1992). Familial heredity factors, prenatal difficulties, and obstetrical complications (Cantwell, 1975; Omenn, 1973; Ross & Ross, 1982) have been reported as possible predisposing factors, as well as selected chromosomal abnormalities (e.g., fragile X). Environmental factors, such as lead poisoning (David, Clark, & Voeller, 1972), refined sugars (Feingold, 1975), allergens (Marshall, 1989), and elevated blood levels (David, Clark, & Hoffman, 1979) also have been asserted as possible etiological agents. Most of these possible causes have received some support in the literature; however, the results have been equivocal.

A neurological etiology for the myriad of behavioral symptoms in ADHD currently has received a fair amount of support in the literature. Impairment in the cortical and subcortical areas of the brain have been reported, with a particular emphasis being placed on possible frontal lobe dysfunction (Lou, Hendriksen, & Bruhn, 1984; Lou, Hendriksen, Bruhn, Borner, & Nielsen, 1989; Chelune, Ferguson, Koon & Dickey,

1986; Grodinsky, 1990; Mariani, 1990). Relatedly, Anastopoulos and Barkley (1988) report findings implicating certain frontal cortical and subcortical areas, in particular the orbital-frontal zone and its connections with the caudate nucleus of the brain. Other specific findings include neurochemical imbalances and/or differences, particularly involving dopamine and norepinephrine, which may be playing a causal role (Zametkin & Rapoport, 1986).

ASSESSMENT STRATEGIES AND CLINICAL ISSUES

To evaluate children with cognitive impairments successfully, certain assessment strategies may be necessary to elicit a child's cooperation, maintain attention, and increase motivation to show their optimal performance. Some strategies may be applicable to all children, although other strategies may be specific to children with particular disabilities. The examiner should keep in mind the type of disorder and the child's level of functioning. The following guidelines, or "rules-of-thumb," can assist professionals who are exposed to children with cognitive disabilities. Although these "rules-of-thumb" are not meant to be exhaustive, they should serve as constants for work with all children.

First, it is important for professionals to remember that cognition cannot and should not be characterized as a unidimensional construct. Although single test scores, such as IQ scores or mental ages, may be useful in beginning to describe a child's level of function, such tools will be woefully inadequate for describing the child's profile of strengths and weaknesses.

Second, given a multidimensional conceptualization of cognition, it becomes paramount for professionals to search during assessment for areas of strength as well as areas of deficit. By uncovering both strengths and weaknesses in a child's cognitive profile, the professional can make better decisions about treatment directions and efforts.

Third, for all children having any type of neurodevelopmental disorder, it is important to remember that cognitive functioning will not necessarily be uniform across neurodevelopmental domains. For example, the professional should attempt to obtain a profile of strengths and weaknesses in the child with mental retardation, though traditional assessment techniques (e.g., intelligence tests) may not be helpful. In these situations it is paramount that the professional utilize other, perhaps informal, assessment strategies to develop this profile. All children with mental retardation or pervasive developmental disorder will not manifest uniformly developed or deficient abilities.

Fourth, it is important for professionals to be hypervigilant on the possible developmental level of the child with whom they are working. For example, when assessing an 8-year-old with moderate mental retardation whose behavior is more characteristic of a 2- to 3-year-old, the examiner should use language that could be understood by a 2-year-old. Conversely, when assessing an 8-year-old with ADHD who is functioning within the average range of intelligence, the examiner may observe behavior that also is characteristic of a 2- to 3-year-old (e.g., tantrums, throwing items, yelling); however, expectations for this child should be consistent with the child's chronological age. This type of professional vigilance facilitates attainment of reliable assessment results.

Fifth, professionals should avoid making "snap" judgments about the overall cognitive level of a child evidencing neurodevelopmental problems. For example, children with learning disabilities typically are viewed by others as "slow" or "lazy," when they may have above average abilities. Such types of "armchair assessments" are insulting to the child and the family, disrespectful to other professionals who may view the child differently, and potentially damaging on how others (e.g., teachers, parents) may work with the child in setting goals and treatment objectives.

Sixth, professionals should be sensitive to the wide array of problems that children with neurocognitive disorders can manifest, particularly social-emotional difficulties. For example, the child with attention deficits may often experience low self-esteem and may show a low frustration tolerance. Although these types of difficulties will not be overcome during an assessment or even following a treatment regimen, professionals who are sensitive to these problems will structure the assessment session for success, provide liberal praise, encouragement, and reinforcement, attempting to work with the child's strengths or what the child can do.

Finally, although it may seem trite, it is important for professionals to treat children with dignity and respect despite the severity of impairment. The professional should call the child by name and not "talk down" to the child. Further, children with autism, mental retardation, or selected types of learning disabilities may have difficulty asking for assistance when it is needed, and the professional should allow time for the child to ask for help before offering it. In addition, the use of reinforcers should be developmentally appropriate, communication should be adapted to the child's behavioral presentation (e.g., simplified language, repetition of one- and two-step commands, the use of nonverbal gestures), and the use of structure and constraints in managing a child's behavior during an assessment should be appropriate to the situation and respectful of parental values.

CONCLUSION

This chapter provided an overview of selected models of cognitive functioning and described the spectrum of cognitive dysfunction in developmental disabilities. We have underscored the general principle that cognitive disorders are most typically mild and diffuse and that associated dysfunctions are the rule rather than the exception. Although this chapter has focused primarily on cognitive dysfunction, the reader will understand that cognitive issues cannot be addressed without consideration of intercurrent primary neurologically based deficits (e.g., motor dysfunction) and primary and/or secondary behaviorally and emotionally based factors to be considered in subsequent chapters.

C H A P T E R   4

CHILDREN WITH SPEECH, LANGUAGE, AND HEARING IMPAIRMENT

Rebecca Landa, Ph.D., CCC-SLP
Michael K. Wynne, Ph.D., CCC-A/SLP

Communication ability impacts many facets of a child's development and functioning. Without it, the world is a mysterious, challenging place. The presence of a communication disorder may impact a child's self-esteem and development in academic, social, and emotional arenas. In many cases, the entire family is affected. To minimize the deleterious effects of a communication disorder, referral to speech-language pathologists and audiologists is necessary for appropriate evaluation and intervention to be provided to the child and family. Diagnostic procedures are available to detect hearing, prespeech, and language abnormalities as early as infancy. Research and clinical experience disproves the wisdom of the "wait and see" stance and the thinking that children cannot be tested before 3 years of age. New research indicates that late talkers are at substantial risk for persisting language deficits that may not be readily detected without appropriate assessment, particularly of certain grammatical language abilities (Paul & Alforde, 1993). This research highlights the importance of involving a speech-language pathologist to provide regular follow-up assessments and, when necessary, communication stimulation programming.

TERMINOLOGY

The term *communication disorder* is a global diagnostic label that indicates abnormality in some aspect of speech and/or language behavior without consideration of etiology. Abnormal communication development has been termed many things, including communication disorder, communication delay, specific language impairment, childhood aphasia or dysphasia, and so on. The diagnosis of communication disorder is made after examination of speech and language abilities relative to each other, as well as to the child's chronological age, cognitive abilities, physiologic capabilities, and cultural background. Children with early speech or language delays are at risk for persistent problems in these areas. Although speech and/or language abnormalities may occur independently of abnormalities in other aspects of development, as pointed out earlier, it is much more common to encounter speech and/or language abnormalities in a setting of associated deficits. When only language abilities are affected (or language deficits are the predominant neurodevelopmental issue), a diagnosis of *specific language impairment* is often given. In a later section of this chapter, this issue will be discussed further.

IDENTIFICATION

Identification of language impairments in children can be a complex process. Motor, auditory, visual, behavioral, socioemotional, attentional, and/or cognitive characteristics of the child may in extreme cases complicate the diagnostic process. The unavailability of standardized tests for assessing some aspects of language development and for assessing adolescent development also contributes to the complexity of diagnosing communication impairments. Diagnoses of speech and language impairments are based on the results of standardized testing, parental report of particular behaviors, structured informal procedures for assessing complex speech and language behaviors for which normed tests are unavailable (e.g., linguistic analyses of language sample data), and behavioral observations (e.g., attention, recall strategies, word retrieval problems, etc.).

Unlike intelligence tests, a single, well-standardized test of language comprehension and expression across the main language domains for a wide age range does not exist. The practice of averaging age-equivalent scores from a number of tests to derive an overall language age equivalency is ill-advised. This is because the psychometric properties, validity, and reliability of individual instruments may vary considerably. Diagnostic batteries must be selected carefully, based on a child's medical, psychiatric, developmental, and educational history, so that complex and subtle impairments can be reliably identified. Children at high risk for language difficulty (e.g., late talkers, siblings of children affected with developmental disorders that seem to be heritable, such as autism, dyslexia, language impairment) should be screened with an appropriate battery at regular intervals because of changes in the nature of disorders for which risk presents at different ages.

HEARING

The inability to hear or process spoken language, even to the mildest degree, can have significant and long-lasting deleterious effects on communicative, social, and academic skills (Maxon & Brackett, 1992). Fortunately, all children are testable with audiologic procedures, as current behavioral and electrophysiological techniques allow audiologists to describe the hearing status of almost any child, regardless of age or disabling condition. The recent draft presenting the proposed revision of the *Joint Committee on Infant Hearing 1990 Position Statement* endorses the concept of universal hearing screening of infants and recommends that this screening be conducted before 3 months of age. Pending development of universal hearing screening programs, the position statement identified various indicators associated with sensorineural and/or conductive hearing loss that can be used to identify those infants who develop health conditions associated with hearing loss and who should receive hearing screening. Table 4–1 presents these indicators.

Hearing screening is often provided during preschool child-find programs and hearing conservation programs offered by public schools and agencies. In addition, many hospitals and private practitioners offer free hearing screenings every May, during Better Speech and Hearing Month. However, whenever the parents or educators of a child suspect hearing difficulties, the child should be referred to an audiologist for hearing screening. Early identification and management of hearing difficulties should be a primary concern for health care professionals. Audiologists and speech-language pathologists are active in developing management programs to promote the functional communication abilities

TABLE 4–1. Various indicators associated with sensorineural and/or conductive hearing loss that can be used to identify infants who develop health conditions associated with hearing loss and should receive hearing screening (Proposed revision of the Joint Committee on Infant Hearing 1990 Position Statement).

A. For use with neonates (birth–28 days) when universal screening is not available.

1. Family history of hereditary childhood sensorineural hearing loss.

2. In utero infection, such as cytomegalovirus, rubella, syphilis, herpes, or toxoplasmosis.

3. Craniofacial anomalies, including those with morphological abnormalities of the pinna and ear canal.

4. Birth weight less than 1500 grams (3.3 lbs.).

5. Hyperbilirubinemia at a serum level requiring exchange transfusion.

6. Ototoxic medications including but not limited to the aminoglycosides used in multiple courses or in combination with loop diuretics.

7. Bacterial meningitis.

8. Severe depression at birth with Apgar scores of 0–4 at one minute or 0–6 at five minutes.

9. Prolonged mechanical ventilation lasting 5 days or longer (e.g., persistent pulmonary hypertension).

10. Stigmata or other findings associated with a syndrome and/or a conductive hearing loss.

B. For use with infants (29 days–2 years) when certain health conditions develop that require re-screening.

1. Parent/caregiver concern regarding hearing, speech, language, and/or developmental delay.

2. Bacterial meningitis and other infections associated with sensorineural hearing loss.

3. Head trauma associated with loss of consciousness or skull fracture.

TABLE 4–1. *(continued)*

4. Stigmata or other findings associated with a syndrome known to include a sensorineural and/or conductive hearing loss.

5. Ototoxic medications including but not limited to chemotherapeutic agents or aminoglycosides used in multiple courses or in combination with loop diuretics.

6. Recurrent or persistent otitis media with effusion for at least 3 months.

C. For use with infants (29 days–3 years) who require periodic monitoring of hearing (indicators associated with delayed onset sensorineural hearing loss):

1. Family history of hereditary childhood hearing loss.

2. In utero infection, such as cytomegalovirus, rubella, syphilis, herpes, or toxoplasmosis.

3. Neurofibromatosis Type II and neurodegenerative disorders.

4. Persistent pulmonary hypertension in the newborn period.

D. For use with infants (29 days–3 years) who require periodic monitoring of hearing (indicators associated with conductive hearing loss):

1. Recurrent or persistent otitis media with effusion.

2. Anatomic deformities and other disorders that affect eustachian tube function.

3. Neurodegenerative disorders.

of children with hearing impairment. Functional communication skills enable children with hearing impairment to understand the information, feelings, and ideas conveyed by family members and friends, as well as to communicate their own thoughts, feelings, and ideas to others.

The impact of a child's hearing impairment is related to the type, severity, and configuration of the hearing loss, as well as the pathology underlying the hearing loss. The time of onset of the hearing difficulties, the stability of the hearing loss, and the progression of the impairment will also influence how a child functions auditorily. In addition, as the ear behaves like a set of narrowly tuned filters or resonance systems, which respond selectively to certain frequencies and attenuate frequencies outside of its acceptance bands (Green, 1976), the frequency selectivity and temporal resolution capabilities of the affected ears will determine how well a child with hearing impairment can process auditory signals when these signals are audible. Finally, the prognosis for the successful habilitation of any hearing impairment is related to the early identification and evaluation of the hearing difficulties and the timely implementation of an appropriate management plan (Diefendorf et al., 1990).

The most common way to describe a child's auditory status is to present the results of an audiological evaluation on an audiogram. An example of an audiogram is presented in Figures 4–1a, b, c. An audiogram provides a graphical representation of the child's thresholds to speech, tonal, and noise stimuli. Frequency (pitch) is represented on the horizontal axis and intensity (loudness) is presented on the vertical axis. Audiologists typically measure hearing sensitivity at octave intervals from 250 Hz to 8000 Hz or roughly from middle C on a piano (C_4 or 262 Hz) to about one octave above the highest note on a piano (C_8 or 4165 Hz). The 0 dB HL line represents the average threshold level for a group of normal hearing young adults with no history of otologic disease or noise exposure.

Although 500, 1000, and 2000 Hz are considered the speech frequencies and define the frequency region containing most of the energy of speech, information about the nature of the speech signal can range from about 100 Hz to 6000 Hz. The intensity scale generally ranges from –10 dB HL to about 120 dB HL. As the intensity scale is on the logarithmic scale, the growth of intensity is not a linear function. Consequently, whispered speech falls between 15 and 20 dB HL, whereas loud speech falls between 60 and 75 dB HL. Most children with normal hearing or with sensorineural hearing loss would find speech uncomfortably loud at about 80 to 90 dB HL. Likewise, speech sounds do not present a uniform spectrum. Vowels tend to have most of their energy in the low to mid frequencies and are produced at relatively higher intensities than consonants. Thus, vowels carry the power of speech. In contrast, consonants tend to have low power and have a significant portion of the frequency spectrum in the higher frequencies. Much of the actual understanding of speech is dependent on the correct perception of the consonants. Consequently, speech may not be audible for children with significant hearing losses across the entire frequency range and speech may be heard but not understood by children with significant hearing losses in the higher frequencies.

A child's hearing impairment can be classified into several different types of hearing losses. Each type of hearing loss may exist in isolation or may be synergistic, with the deleterious effects of each type additive. Typically, the classification is based on the loci of the hearing loss or the site of the lesion within the auditory system. A pure *conductive hearing loss* exists when the sound conducting mechanism is impaired in some aspect. The child has some degree of hearing loss because the signal cannot be transmitted to the inner ear without some increase in intensity. A conductive hearing loss has a strictly peripheral site of lesion, specifically from the opening of the outer ear canal to the membrane covering the oval window of the inner ear, including any abnormalities on the medial wall of the middle ear cavity. Although air-conduction thresholds are poorer than normal in conductive hearing losses, the bone-conduction thresholds must be within the normal limits for hearing sensitivity and should be better than the air-conduction thresholds by at least 15 dB. An audiogram illustrating a conductive hearing loss is presented in Figure 4–1a. Conductive hearing loss accounts for a majority of the pediatric audiologist's case load and is very common in infants and children, particularly because of the prevalence of middle ear infections in this age group. Children with craniofacial anomalies, developmental disabilities, and poorly developed immune systems have a high risk for developing conductive hearing loss. Conductive hearing losses are generally temporary, as most of the pathologies respond to medical treatment.

A pure *sensorineural hearing loss* exists when the sound conducting mechanism is normal in every respect but the child has some loss of hearing sensitivity because the signal cannot be correctly transduced, analyzed, or perceived. The child has some degree of hearing loss because certain characteristics of the signal are not appropriately processed by the inner ear and/or the subsequent neural pathways. When the site of the lesion is located within the cochlea, the hearing loss is from a sensory (end organ) pathology; whereas, when the site of lesion is located within the neural pathways, the hearing loss is caused by retro-cochlear pathology. In sensorineural hearing losses, both the air- and bone-conduction thresholds are poorer than the normal range of hearing sensitivity. An audiogram illustrating a sensorineural hearing loss is presented in Figure 4–1b. As with conductive hearing losses, children with cranial facial anomalies and developmental disabilities have a high risk for having sensorineural hearing losses. In addition, exposure to high noise levels, ototoxic medications, and head trauma can also result in significant sensorineural hearing losses. Generally, sensorineural hearing loss is permanent and rarely can be treated medically. Hearing aids, hearing assistance technologies, and aural habilitation is the preferred course of treatment for children with sensorineural hearing losses. Some children may need to move to manual communication systems such as American Sign Language for the primary language input.

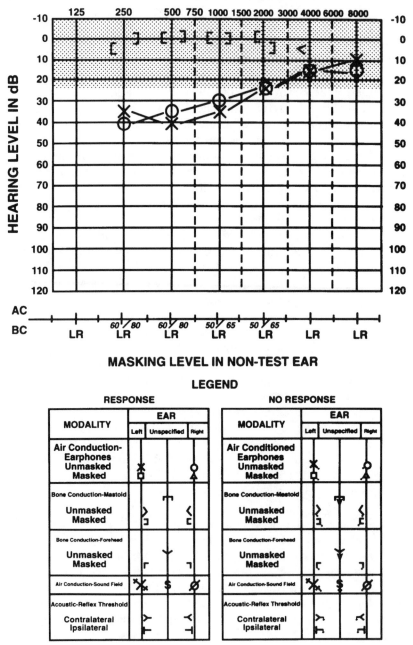

FIGURE 4-1a. Audiogram of a conductive hearing loss.

FREQUENCY IN HERTZ

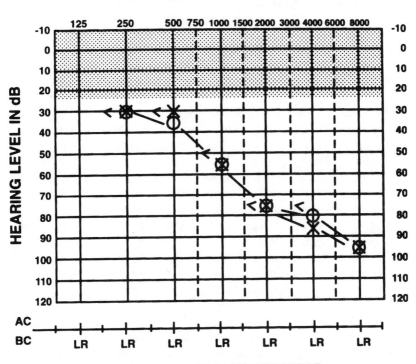

MASKING LEVEL IN NON-TEST EAR

LEGEND

RESPONSE				NO RESPONSE			
MODALITY	**EAR**			**MODALITY**	**EAR**		
	Left	Unspecified	Right		Left	Unspecified	Right
Air Conduction-Earphones Unmasked Masked	✗ □		○ △	**Air Conditioned Earphones** Unmasked Masked	✗ □		○ △
Bone Conduction-Mastoid Unmasked Masked	> ⊐	⌐	< ⊏	Bone Conduction-Mastoid Unmasked Masked	⋗	⫪	⋖
Bone Conduction-Forehead Unmasked Masked	⌐	⋎	⌐	Bone Conduction-Forehead Unmasked Masked	⌐	⋎	⌐
Air Conduction-Sound Field	✗	$	∅	Air Conduction-Sound Field	✗	$	∅
Acoustic-Reflex Threshold Contralateral Ipsilateral	⊱ ⊥		⊰ ⊤	Acoustic-Reflex Threshold Contralateral Ipsilateral	⊱ ⊥		⊰ ⊤

FIGURE 4–1b. Audiogram of a sensorineural hearing loss.

93

A *mixed hearing loss* exists when both conductive and sensorineural hearing losses are present in the same ear. In this type of hearing loss, both lesions are additive resulting in significant air-bone gaps, with the bone-conduction thresholds falling outside the normal range of hearing sensitivity. An audiogram illustrating a mixed hearing loss is presented in Figure 4–1c. In most cases, both medical and audiological management programs are needed to address the health and communication needs of the child.

In addition to these traditional types of hearing loss, many children present with *central auditory processing disorders* (Gravel & Stapells, 1993; Hall et al., 1993; Stach & Loiselle, 1993). A pure central auditory processing disorder exists when hearing sensitivity is normal but the child fails to perceive and use acoustic information because the central auditory system is unable to appropriately process the signals transduced by the cochlea. Despite having normal hearing acuity, children with auditory processing disorders may exhibit delayed and/ or disordered listening behaviors because of their difficulties processing acoustic signals (Wynne, 1992). Children who present with central auditory processing disorders are often taught compensation strategies and receive extensive auditory training to improve their ability to comprehend speech in critical listening situations. Recent studies by Jerger and colleagues (Jerger, 1992; Jerger & Chmiel, 1993; Jerger, Oliver, & Martin, 1990) have also indicated that many adults with sensorineural hearing losses have concomitant central auditory processing disorders, often confounding the evaluation and successful management of the sensorineural hearing loss. Although there is no empirical evidence to prove the existence of central auditory processing difficulties in children with sensorineural hearing loss, clinical experience suggests that this is, indeed, the case.

The severity and configuration of a hearing loss not only helps determine the nature of the pathology but often determines the nature and course of management. Table 4–2 presents the range and effects of the various degrees of hearing loss (Anderson, 1991). Although the percentage of hearing loss can be determined for medical-legal purposes, the *degree* of hearing loss cannot be defined as a percentage, because the effects of the loss are dependent on both the severity and configuration of the hearing loss. A mild rising hearing loss and a mild sloping hearing loss may have equivalent percentage of hearing loss, yet have quite different effects on a child's communication skills and management plan.

The temporal characteristics of the hearing loss also contribute to the child's communication difficulties. Generally, the effects of hearing loss are greater with its earlier onset, particularly if the hearing loss

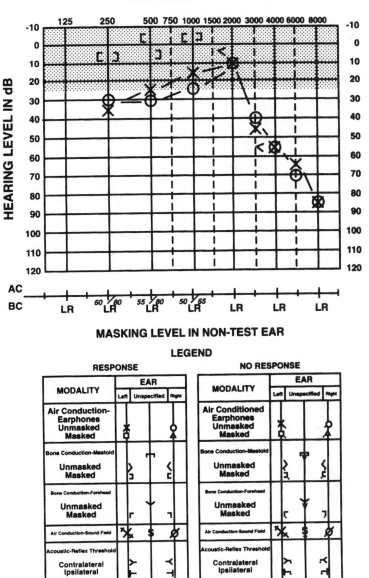

FIGURE 4–1c. Audiogram of a mixed hearing loss.

is prelinguistic (before the development of language). Furthermore, the identification and management of a childhood hearing loss is much more difficult if the hearing loss is fluctuating or progressive. Because

TABLE 4–2. Possible effects of hearing loss of increasing degree.

Degree of Hearing Loss	Severity	Possible Effects	Possible Educational Needs
-10 to 15 db HL	Normal	None	None
16 to 25 dB HL	Slight	The child may have difficulties hearing faint speech, especially in difficult listening situations. The child may be unaware of subtle conversational cues which could cause some inappropriate behavior. The child may be more fatigued due to increased listening effort.	The child will benefit from preferential seating and possible from routine medical and/or audiological monitoring. The child may benefit from mild gain hearing assistance technologies. The child may require speech-language services.
26 to 40 dB HL	Mild	At 30 dB, a child can miss between 25–40% of the speech signal. In difficult listening environments, up to 50% of the primary speech signal may be missed. The child may not attend to speech and become easily fatigued because of increased listening effort.	The child will benefit from amplification and hearing assistance technologies. The child may need additional educational services to address any deficits in their speech-language skills and in their academic performance. Teacher in-service is strongly recommended.
41 to 55 dB HL	Moderate	The child likely understands conversational speech only at a close distance, in a clear and distinct manner, and	Amplification and hearing assistance technology are essential in the classroom. The child will likely benefit from

TABLE 4-2 *(continued)*

Degree of Hearing Loss	Severity	Possible Effects	Possible Educational Needs
		in a favorable listening situation. The hearing loss will likely have some effect on the child's speech and language skills as well as on academic performance.	additional educational services to address any deficits in their speech-language skills and in academic performance. Teacher in-service is strongly recommended.
56 to 70 dB HL	Moderate to Severe	Without amplification, conversational speech is very difficult to hear. The child will have some delayed or disordered speech and language skills. Needing to constantly wear hearing aids, the child is perceived as a special learner.	Full-time amplification is required and hearing assistance technologies are essential in the classroom. The child will likely require additional educational services to address any deficits in speech-language skills and in academic performance. Teacher in-service is necessary.
71 to 90 dB HL	Severe	Without amplification, speech must be very loud if it is to be heard. Even when aided, the child may have significant difficulties hearing and understanding speech. The child will have some delayed or disordered speech and language skills.	In addition to the communication and educational needs above, the child may require the use of a sign language system as part of an overall communication program.

(continued)

TABLE 4–2 (*continued*)

Degree of Hearing Loss	Severity	Possible Effects	Possible Educational Needs
		Needing to constantly wear hearing aids, the child is perceived as a special learner.	
>90 dB HL	Profound	Even when aided with conventional hearing aids, speech is very difficult to understand. In many cases, the child may only be aware of sound and not appropriately perceive it. The child will likely rely on visual cues to communicate effectively.	In addition to the communication described above, the child may require cochlear implants or tactile aids to perceive the acoustic cues of speech. Some families may choose a bilingual, bicultural approach to language development.

Modified from Anderson (1991).

of the dynamic nature of hearing status in infants and young children, a single evaluation provides a static profile of the hearing loss and may not yield sufficient diagnostic results to adequately address the medical and habilitative needs of the infant or toddler with hearing impairment. Periodic and, in some cases, frequent hearing evaluations are needed to fully define the status of the auditory system of a child with hearing impairment and how to best remediate any hearing difficulties. Furthermore, simply because an infant or child passed a hearing screening in the past does not rule out hearing difficulties in the present.

The assessment of the auditory system in infants and children is accomplished by immittance, electrophysiological, and/or behavioral measures. *Tympanometry*, the most frequently used immittance measure to assess the status of the conductive mechanism in children, consists of measuring the impedance of the tympanic membrane for the transmission of a tone. Using a nominal 220 Hz probe tone, immittance audiometers measure the amount of sound reflected off the tympanic membrane through changes in pressure. Although tympanometry is sensitive to middle ear pathologies affecting the tympanic membrane at all ages, it lacks specificity for infants younger than 6 months of age because of the high compliance of their external ear canal walls (Nozza, Bluestone, Kardatzke & Bachman, 1992).

Physiological measures consist of *Brain stem-evoked response* (BSER) audiometry and *otoacoustic emission* (OAE) testing (Bess, 1993; Picton, 1992). These measures can detect and, in some cases, provide excellent estimates of hearing loss in infants and older children who are unable to respond reliably to behavioral measures of hearing sensitivity. BSER audiometry measures the electrical potentials generated by the nerves within the VIIIth cranial nerve and lower auditory brain stem to rapid-onset, short-duration acoustic signals such as a click stimulus. Because these signals are very quiet and are buried in a large amount of noise, signal-averaging techniques are used to record the electrical response of the auditory system. The response is judged by the presence of a positive wavelet, typically wave V, occurring within a certain latency range. The latencies, amplitudes, and morphologies of the responses are dependent on the child's age, the stimulus characteristics, and the recording parameters; however, individuals with normal peripheral ear and lower auditory brain stem system integrity will demonstrate a response to clicks at intensities down to 30 dB HL. Under most stimulus conditions, the response is sensitive to the hearing status between 2000 and 4000 Hz (Gravel & Stapells, 1993). Although different methods of evoked-potential testing can estimate hearing sensitivity outside this frequency range, that testing is more difficult and the results have less reliability.

OAE testing is a relatively new means of detecting hearing loss in infants and children (Kemp & Ryan, 1993; Norton, 1993; White, Vohr, & Behrens, 1993). The cochlea will generate a low-intensity acoustic echo in response to an auditory stimulus in individuals with normal activity of the outer hair cells, who present normal conductive mechanisms. There also appears to be a developmental change in the nature of evoked otoacoustic emissions, as infants and young children demonstrate much larger emissions than do adults. Hearing losses from cochlear and/or middle ear pathologies can be readily identified using OAEs; however, these measurements generally fail to define the severity of the hearing loss. Although there are four different types of otoacoustic emissions, *transient-evoked otoacoustic emissions* (TEOAEs) and *distortion product otoacoustic emissions* (DPOAEs) are the preferred types of emissions used to identify hearing loss in infants and children. Other methods are also available for testing infants and children. The skilled pediatric audiologist will select appropriate measures for each child, adjusting for the strengths and weaknesses of each approach.

Pediatric audiology is a dynamic process and each audiological evaluation should lead to an appropriate and comprehensive management plan. Children with conductive and mixed hearing loss should receive medical treatment and monitoring to address the pathologies affecting the transmission of the signal to the inner ear. A percentage of these children may also be candidates for amplification (hearing aids), depending on the nature of the conductive component causing their hearing difficulties.

Aural (re)habilitation programs for children with sensorineural components to their hearing difficulties generally include amplification (hearing aids), hearing assistance technologies such as FM systems, auditory training, and speech-language remediation. Hearing aids are imperfect devices fitted to impaired ears and simply do not resolve all of the hearing difficulties faced by children with hearing impairment. The successful fit and use of hearing aids and hearing assistance technologies are paramount for communication development in most children with sensorineural hearing loss (Maxon & Smaldino, 1991). Just like any other mechanical and electrical device, hearing aids will break down. Consequently, it is imperative that someone performs a daily listening check on hearing aids to ensure that units are working appropriately. For those children who are unable to obtain any real benefit from conventional hearing aids, cochlear implants become a viable option. These surgical implants deliver an electrical signal to viable auditory nerve fibers and have proven to be very effective in addressing the hearing needs of many children who are deaf.

Parents of children with educationally significant hearing losses also may choose to use sign language systems as a primary component of the management program. Using a sign language system as a component of the management program does not mean that the child should not receive additional assistance in the development of their speech and oral language skills. Children with even mild hearing losses may require speech-language therapy to obtain functional communication skills (Gordon-Brannan, Hodson, & Wynne, 1992). Many individuals who are deaf advocate a bilingual, bicultural approach for the language development in children who cannot hear. Regardless of the bias of physicians, educators, advocates, speech-language pathologists, and audiologists, parents have the responsibility to choose the communication mode and management plan that they believe will best serve the needs of their child. They should receive unbiased information on all of the management and educational options available to their family. Finally, once they have selected a management plan, the family should be encouraged to actively participate in the habilitation process, while having the freedom to change the management plan any time during the course of treatment.

OVERVIEW OF SPEECH SYSTEMS

The act of speaking is multifaceted and requires, in part, intact coordination and structure of respiratory, laryngeal, and oral (articulation and resonation) systems. These systems serve to generate and valve the airstream in all the ways necessary to produce the speech sounds of a language. In typical individuals, the respiratory and laryngeal systems act in synchrony, with air being pushed from the lungs, through the trachea and larynx. Rapid opening and closing of the vocal folds within the larynx produces the primary vibration in the airstream needed to produced vocalizations. The resulting rather undifferentiated glottal tone is transformed into meaningful speech by modification of the acoustic properties of the pharyngeal, oral, and nasal cavities. Such modification is achieved by movements of the articulators (tongue, palate, lips, and jaw), which change the resonance characteristics of these cavities. A disruption in any of the above systems will affect speech production.

The speech systems come under increasing voluntary control and coordination until adolescence. Progressively, infants become able to isolate movements in the articulators and to coordinate these movements with respiratory and laryngeal action to mark the prosodic features of rhythm, stress, intonation, and rate that augment the linguistic content of speech in important ways. (See Prosody section below.) Gradually, infantile temporal patterning, resonance, and acoustic characteristics give way to a more adult-like speech quality allowed by changes in neuromotor control coupled with changes in size and shape of the vocal tract. Below, some disorders associated with each speech system are described. For the articulatory system, for which definable stages of development occur, the developmental process is also briefly reviewed.

The Respiratory System

The respiratory system for speech is controlled by neurons in the anterior horns of the thoracic and cervical spinal cord, with some involvement of the XIth cranial nerve. This widespread arrangement leads to a variety of clinical symptoms when impairment occurs. For example, abnormal breathing patterns may result from inadequate or reduced respiratory support for speech secondary to muscle weakness, abnormal muscle tone, or incoordination. These problems may be seen in children with cerebral palsy, cerebrovascular accident and trauma, and in the later stages of neurodegenerative diseases. Patients with these disorders may adopt an abnormal pattern of breathing, with extreme tension in the neck, laryngeal, and facial regions. This results in a voice disorder, characterized by a harsh, high-pitched voice with inadequate loudness and pitch variation. Many children with cerebral palsy exhibit rapid and shallow inhalation, poorly controlled exhalation, involuntary movements in the respiratory musculature, and antagonistic diaphragmatic-abdominal and thoracic movements. This leads to voice and speech abnormalities.

The Laryngeal System

Laryngeal abnormalities resulting in voice disorders occur in 3 to 5% of school-age children. Typically, abnormal voice quality (voice disorder) results from mass/size changes in the vocal folds, incomplete closure of the vocal folds, or asymmetry in vocal fold motion. These problems may result from: (1) functional causes, such as speaking at an inappropriate pitch (causing nodules), or (2) organic causes such as allergy (causing edema of laryngeal tissue), structural abnormalities (e.g., juvenile papillomata, vocal web, polyps), or neurophysiologic abnormality (vocal fold paralysis). The diagnosis and treatment of voice disorders involves both medical and speech-language professionals. Assessment must include a careful analysis of medical and neurological factors, including a history of vocal use, careful documentation of alterations in quality, pitch, and loudness of the voice, and an examination of laryngeal anatomy and function through direct or indirect laryngoscopy.

The Resonance System

Perception of normal resonance depends on the volume, shape, and surfaces of the vocal tract structures, the size of the mouth opening, and the occlusion of the nasal cavity. Abnormalities in any of these may result in impaired vowel production, hypernasality, or hyponasality. Resonance problems may be associated with hearing loss, physiologic problems because of a lesion of the central nervous system, or anatomic defects of the orofacial region.

In individuals who are deaf, resonance abnormality may be related to problems learning proper control of nasal coupling because of (1) the invisibility of the raising and lowering palate during speech not being detectable by lip reading and (2) the limited proprioceptive feedback provided during velopharyngeal closure. Thus, a child who is deaf has difficulty self-monitoring resonance patterns. Some physiologic defects leading to abnormal resonance include the dysarthrias, acute myopathies, and peripheral neuropathologies. Resonance abnormalities associated with the dysarthrias result from abnormal tongue positioning, inappropriate degree of tension in the speech musculature, and inappropriate closure of the velopharyngeal opening. The more common anatomic defects include orofacial clefts, cleft lip, and cleft palate, which occur in 700 to 800 babies per year in the United States of America.

Hypernasality, with or without audible nasal emission of air, is the result of an inadequately occluded nasal cavity during the articulation of nonnasal speech sounds (all vowels and consonants except for *m, n, ng*). Hypernasality is not only socially challenging for the child, but may also lead to problems of poor speech intelligibility from subsequent articulatory, phonatory, and prosodic problems caused by a poorly valved airstream. Children with short velums or minimal or inefficient pharyngeal wall movement should be carefully evaluated before adenoids are removed. Such tissue may serve to assist in occluding the nasal cavity for these children. In some cases, a severe hypernasality may occur once the nasal-occluding assistance of adenoidal tissue is removed.

Hyponasality results from failure of sound to enter the nasal cavity during articulation of the nasal consonants. This may result from anatomic problems (e.g., obstruction of the nasal passageways or nasopharyngeal space) and/or poor timing of velopharyngeal closure (as seen in individuals who are deaf). Referral to an otolaryngologist is necessary in most cases of hyponasality to diagnose and treat possible obstruction of the nasal cavity.

The Articulatory System

Articulation involves mastery of the motor ability to produce the sounds and sound sequences of a language. For example, the child must learn to control: air flow from the lungs through the larynx, vocal fold movement for the production of voiced and voiceless consonants (e.g., *b* versus *p*), the opening and closing of the velopharyngeal mechanism to produce nasal and oral sounds (e.g., *n* versus *d*), and so on. In addition to this, the child must learn that the production of contrasts such as voiced-voiceless and nasal-oral have meaning, communicating differences in words such as *Ben* versus *pen* and *no* versus *doe*. Correct articulation also depends on knowledge of the phonological rules of the language. These rules involve learning: (1) which sounds are used in the language to create meaningful words (e.g., *r* and *l* are separate contrastive sounds in English but not in Chinese), (2) the constraints of sound sequences for the language (e.g., the *ng* sound is never used at the beginning of a word in English), and (3) how sound production changes in connected speech and when grammatical markers are added (e.g., the *t* in *hit* is pronounced differently when it precedes an unstressed vowel as in *hitter*).

The precursors to articulation develop during infancy in a series of well-defined stages, which are related to each other hierarchically (Oller, 1980; Stark, 1980). The first of these stages, the reflexive stage (0–2 months), is characterized by crying and vegetative sounds (e.g., burping, sneezing). The vocal repertoire is increased with the addition of open sounds, or vowels, and with the discontinuation of obligatory nasal breathing. This milestone marks the onset of the cooing stage (2–3 months). At the "expansion" stage (4–5 months), an increase occurs in the variety of sounds produced, with squeals and raspberries emerging. During the marginal babbling stage (6–8 months), the combination of consonant-like and vowel-like sounds occurs, with the timing characteristics of these sounds differing from those of meaningful speech. Between 9 and 12 months, infants produce strings of identifiable syllables known as reduplicative babbling (e.g., "bababable"). These productions are thought to form the basis for meaningful speech. At the second expansion stage (12–18 months), the ability to produce different sound combinations rather than repetition of the same consonant-vowel sequence emerges (e.g., "badibega"). New intonation patterns also emerge during this stage, giving the babbling a speech-like pattern. Although many skills build on related rudimentary skills in previous stages, new behaviors also emerge that appear to be unrelated to previously developed skills (Stark, 1980).

Variability in control of the speech mechanism decreases as neuromotor control increases, with control being fairly well established by 3 or 4 years of age. Between 8 and 12 years of age, control of the speech mechanism has reached full maturity (Kent, 1976). The sequence in which speech sounds are mastered is fairly predictable, based on the motoric complexity involved in the articulation of the speech sound.

Articulation disorders occur in about 10% of kindergarten and first grade children, gradually declining in frequency thereafter. Rarely, articulation problems persist into adulthood. Problems with articulation occur more often in males than in females. Articulation errors have traditionally been defined as omission, substitution, distortion, or addition of a sound or sounds. Evaluation of articulation disorders includes examination of type, number, frequency, consistency, and pattern of errors. The degree to which the child is able to approximate correct production of speech sounds and with what type and degree of assistance from the speech-language pathologist is also examined.

Articulation disorders are sometimes associated with obvious structural anomalies, as in cleft palate, severe malocclusion, macroglossia and other abnormalities of the tongue, neurologic impairment as in the dysarthrias, or sensory deficits as in hearing impairment. In most cases, the etiology of the articulation problem is not clear. Developmental apraxia may be diagnosed when children exhibit multiple articulation errors with little response to traditional articulation treatment. This disorder affects the coordination of movements of the respiratory, laryngeal, and oral musculature in articulation. Authorities (Haynes, 1985) on this disorder believe that impairment occurs in the motor planning stage of speech production. Typically, children thought to have developmental apraxia of speech exhibit a restricted repertoire of speech sounds, inability to produce speech sounds requiring complex articulatory adjustments (e.g., *sh*, *f*), variable articulation of speech sounds, vowel and consonant errors, and prosodic abnormalities involving a slowed rate and monotony of stress patterns.

In some cases, articulation disorders actually reflect a linguistic impairment. This is determined through a phonological analysis, which involves examining errors across phonetic contexts and determining the types of underlying rules that predict the errors produced by the child. For example, one type of phonological process that could result in mispronounced words is that of *fronting* (Ingram, 1976). This process involves producing a speech sound more toward the front of the oral cavity than is appropriate. This is seen when the *k* and *g* sounds are systematically produced as *t* and *d*, respectively. Here, sounds that should have been produced with the back of the tongue against the back portion of the palate are produced with the tongue tip toward the front of the mouth.

The nature of the treatment program recommended for articulation disorders will depend on the nature and severity of the errors as well as the presence of motor, cognitive, social, and language difficulties. For children who are unable to speak or whose speech is unintelligible, a supplemental or augmentative communication system may be prescribed by the speech-language pathologist. These systems range in the degree of abstraction of the symbols employed (from real objects to letters) and in the degree of technological sophistication (from gaze systems and picture boards to sophisticated computerized devices with speech output).

Prosody

Prosody of speech consists of rhythm, stress, intonation, and rate. These features of speech are produced by variations in pitch, loudness, articulatory speed, and pause time. Prosody of speech communicates much information about the attitudes and intentions of the speaker. It also contributes to the meaning of an utterance. Prosodic cues direct the listener's attention to the most salient aspects of a message. For example, the sentence, "I am here," may be used to express a number of different meanings. Prosodic cues will indicate whether the intended meaning is: (a) I, not Bob, am here; (b) I am here, not there; (c) I am not absent as was just stated by someone else. Prosody is abnormal in the speech of those who are deaf, persons who have dysarthria, and in developmental apraxia of speech. Perception and production of prosody may also be abnormal in some persons who are language disordered, autistic, head-injured, mentally retarded, and otherwise impaired.

Fluency

Fluency disorders, often referred to as *stuttering*, are typically characterized by repetition of speech sounds or syllables or blockage of articulation or vocalization. Some individuals develop reactions (secondary behaviors) to these speech difficulties as they struggle to overcome the initial difficulty. These behaviors may manifest as movement of other body parts before or during speech.

Fluency disruptions are most commonly seen between 2 and 5 years of age. Early intervention greatly improves prognosis and decreases the likelihood that complicating secondary behaviors will develop. Signs that a referral is appropriate include:

1. Child is aware that a problem exists.
2. Marked tension and audible or visible signs of struggle are present during speech.
3. The speech pattern attracts attention to itself or interferes with communication.
4. Speech is characterized by sound prolongations (especially with pitch changes), syllable or word repetitions (especially when there are rate variations), or pauses within words, before speaking or after the dysfluency.
5. Child avoids certain words or sounds.
6. Parent speaks for child when communicative difficulty is present or parent frequently interrupts child.
7. Parents are concerned about the way the child speaks or about the child's reaction to the dysfluencies.
8. Frequent reformulation (rewording) of a sentence before it is completed.

An interaction of environmental and biological factors appear to contribute to the onset of stuttering. Stutterers tend to exhibit speech motor, central auditory processing, and language impairment in childhood. As a group, they are slow to achieve language milestones and exhibit more frequent articulation difficulties than children who do not stutter. Although the incidence of stuttering is greater in males than in females, severity of dysfluency may be greater in affected females than in males. Electrophysiologic and behavioral research are adding to our understanding of this complex disorder.

It is clear that social stress exacerbates dysfluency and that rhythmic, structured speaking situations often facilitate fluent speech. Intervention must incorporate a variety of techniques, addressing social, psychological, speech planning, and language domains. For maximal success, it is important for family members to be involved in the treatment process.

Some fluency problems may be quite severe but differ qualitatively from stuttering. Nonstuttering dysfluency is sometimes characterized by multiple attempts at wording a sentence before actually completing the sentence. By the time the child completes the sentence, the listener may not be sure what the child was communicating. School-age children with this problem may have difficulty giving a well-organized and coherent account of an event or story. Such problems may be related to planning messages on an ideational level, word finding problems, linguistic organization, or some other difficulty.

LANGUAGE

Language is a multidimensional phenomenon. It may be conceptualized as having four interdependent yet theoretically distinct subsystems. These are phonology, grammar (morphology and syntax), semantics, and pragmatics. Phonology pertains to linguistic rules affecting speech and has been referred to in the section on speech production. The remaining three subsystems are described, followed by a brief description of normal development in that area. Although general milestones are provided below for each language domain, there is strong evidence for at least two different patterns of language development (see Bates, Bretherton, & Snyder, 1988, for a review).

Grammatical Development

Learning grammatical rules allows children to properly arrange grammatical markers (e.g., verb tense markers such as -ed, plural markers such as *s*) and word sequences for sentence formation. Children learn that meaningful relationships are conveyed by the way in which words are ordered and combined. They come to know that the sentences "Sue hit Bob" and "Bob hit Sue" contain the same words but do not convey the same meaning. Knowledge of grammatical rules allows children to recognize that if Bob did the hitting, his name must precede the verb unless there are other grammatical markers present that indicate otherwise. For example, when the grammatical marker "was" precedes an uninflected verb and the verb is followed by the marker "by," as in the sentence "Sue was hit by Bob," the listener knows that the first person mentioned was the recipient of the action, not the actor.

The onset of grammatical development may occur as early as 16 months, with a spurt in grammatical development occurring between 20 and 36 months of age. This is the time when word combinations are used to express relationships between people, events, and objects. Early grammatical structures are very simple, usually taking the form of noun + noun (e.g., "Daddy car), noun + verb (e.g., Car go), verb + noun (e.g., "Gimme cookie"), or adjective + noun (e.g., "big ball"). This early stage of grammatical development is often described as "telegraphic" because the short, simple nature of the sentences resembles a telegram. These short sentences are primarily made up of words such as nouns and verbs that are rich in semantic content, or meaning. Other types of words ("function words" such as prepositions, conjunctions, and articles) tend to be lacking. The types of words used in early sentences and the average length of these sentences may serve as indications of how normally a child's early grammatical system is developing.

Gradually, the grammatical rule system becomes more complex. Grammatical markers are added to sentences in a predictable order: first the *ing* verb marker, then the plural *s*, and so on (Brown, 1973). Noun and verb phrases become elaborated, enabling a child to express increasing amounts of information within a sentence. Rules are learned for embedding one sentence within another, resulting in an elaborate, complex sentence such as, "The boy who is sitting under the tree is eating apples." Rules for changing one type of sentence into another are also learned. For example, declarative sentences such as "Bob hit Sue" may be changed into negative sentences ("Bob did not hit Sue") or into interrogative sentences ("Did Bob hit Sue?"). This flexibility is critical if a child is to express meaning accurately and in socially acceptable ways.

Although the basic structures of grammar are learned before 4 years of age, some significant changes occur in grammatical development after this age. Between 4 and 6 years, children shift from an "intrasentential grammar" (grammar used to express simple meanings within a sentence) to "intersentential grammar" (grammar used to express relationships between sentences). That is, grammar is used to make discourse cohesive and coherent. For example, words such as pronouns (e.g., *he*) must be clearly referenced first so that speaker and listener share the same information. Acquiring this use of grammar is closely tied to the development of social cognition, especially the ability to appreciate others' perspectives. During adolescence, syntactic skills continue to develop. For example, noun phrase postmodification becomes more complex through the use of a variety of syntactic mechanisms. In the following sentence, the noun "air" is postmodified by the prepositional phrase "in the mountains": "I saw that the air *in the mountains* goes down and heats off" (Scott, 1988, p.64). Other changes occur gradually over time, with increasing use of complex forms and development of skill in the grammar of expository text.

One misconception about grammatical skill is that comprehension precedes production—such that if a child is able to produce a grammatical structure, the youngster must comprehend that structure. However, children sometimes produce complex forms or sentence structures for which they have not mastered the grammatical rules and that they may not understand. This is possible because of a number of tacit strategies that children use. For example, children may store in memory multiword units that are, in the mind of the child, a sort of "giant" word (e.g., "gimme that"). In this case, the child does not realize the power of the words in that sentence to be rearranged and combined with other words in the youngster's vocabulary and, therefore, is restricted in the ability to express ideas in the most socially acceptable or most efficient way. Another possible explanation is that children repeat or build upon an utterance produced earlier in the conversation, either by him or herself or the conversational partner. For example, the mother might say, "Does Mike want his ball?" and the child might say, "Mike want ball." This child may not go on to form sentences such as "I want cookie," or "I want a ride," or " I want mom," despite having the vocabulary to do so (Coggins & Carpenter, 1979). To determine whether the utterances produced by a child are rule-based or strategy-based and if utterances are developmentally appropriate, a careful grammatical analysis of an extended language sample is necessary.

Semantic Development

Semantic knowledge encompasses information about word meaning (lexical semantics) and how word meanings relate to each other (relational semantics). Knowledge of relational semantics enables the child to recognize that the grammatically intact sentence, "Colorless green ideas sleep furiously" is meaningless. Such knowledge also enables a child to recognize the dual meaning of the sentence "Flying planes can be dangerous."

Semantic development is closely tied to a child's conceptual development. Assessment of semantic knowledge is a multifaceted process that is not adequately accomplished by administering verbal subtests of an intelligence test or a test of single-word vocabulary comprehension such as the *Peabody Picture Vocabulary Test-Revised (PPVT-R)* (Dunn & Dunn, 1981). Speech-language pathologists assess semantic development using standardized and nonstandardized protocols to examine comprehension and production of abstract concepts, relational terms, multiple-meaning words (e.g., run) and sentences, figurative language, humor, inferential skills, word retrieval, and so on. Such assessment enables the speech-language pathologist to determine if there is a semantic impairment and how the semantic subsystem is developing relative to other language subsystems.

Comprehension of words is seen toward the end of the first year of life, with words representing what children learn about people, events, objects, and relationships being the first to enter the child's mental dictionary. Children's ideas about a word's meaning may be somewhat unstable at that time. Thus, comprehension is most facilitated within familiar routines and with the provision of cues (e.g., pointing). Between 12 and 18 months of age, children's comprehension of words or phrases is best observed within interaction routines rather than when asked to point to one of two pictures named by an examiner. At that age, responsiveness to spoken language varies with attention, interest, familiarity, comfort level, context, and complexity of the verbal input.

Comprehension of language gradually becomes less dependent on contextual cues and routines. Between 16 and 18 months, comprehension of novel word combinations (e.g., "kiss the car") emerges. Comprehension of longer word combinations, more complex meaning relationships (e.g., time and kinship relationships), multiple-sentence input as occurs in stories or conversation, words with multiple meanings, and so on emerges throughout childhood and adolescence. Most first graders demonstrate metalinguistic knowledge, which enables them to think about language explicitly and to consider the structural properties of language. Such ability is necessary to identify the "sounds" making up a word, to identify the "words" in a "sentence," write "sentences," and so on. By 9 years of age, basic comprehension of various types of figurative language (e.g., idioms, proverbs, metaphor, etc.) is achieved, but continued development in lexical and syntactic areas, analytical reasoning, and world knowledge facilitate the ever-increasing competence with this facet of language (Nippold, 1988). The acquisition of the knowledge discussed above sets the stage for success with the language of learning, integrating information presented in books or conversations, and understanding the humor and figures of speech used by peers, which is important for peer acceptance and academic success.

Production of first words typically occurs between 12 and 18 months. However, the child's mental dictionary at this stage does not parallel that of the adult. Although the specific words acquired will differ from child to child, the general types of concepts represented by those words are rather predictable. The words usually represent a person, object, or event salient to the child, or something dynamic that directly impacts the child. Thus, the word "ball," which the child may act on and has interesting motion patterns is likely to be acquired before the word "wall," which is static and has less relevance to the child. Early conceptualization of a word's meaning is typically more general or restricted than the adult definition of the word. This is typically a very short-lived phenomenon. The ability to actually define a word does not emerge until the late preschool years.

When children begin to produce 50–75 words (around 18 months of age), a rapid surge in vocabulary development typically occurs, in which 300 words might be added to an expressive vocabulary in 6 months. This surge is accompanied by a change in vocabulary composition, with a proportional increase in verbs, adjectives, and other words that play a relational role in the language. According to Bates, Thal, and Janowsky (1992), this change may represent a shift from using words primarily to reference things (at the single word stage) to serving a predication role (relational meaning in word combinations). This is the stage when word combinations begin to appear (18–20 months). According to Bates et al. (1992), the primary meaning relationships produced at this stage (regardless of native language) involve expression of existence (e.g., appearance, disappearance, and reappearance of interesting objects), desires (e.g., refusal, denial, requests), event relations (possession, agent-action-object, change of state or location), and attribution (e.g., "hot, big"). With increasing conceptual and memory capacity, children begin to express multiple meaning relationships within one utterance and to express increasingly complex relationships. By first grade, many children are able to create sequenced stories with meaningful plots and characters.

Pragmatic Development

Pragmatic development encompasses a range of skills central to the social use of language, representing an integration of affective, social, cognitive, and linguistic knowledge. This process begins very early in life, with prelinguistic behaviors such as eye contact, affective reciprocity, social smile, vocal turn-taking, and anticipatory gestures. Abnormalities in these early behaviors are a red flag that problems may appear in the future. When intentional communication appears (9–12 months), gestures, vocalizations, and words are used for a variety of social (greeting, showing, commenting) and regulatory (requesting, protesting) functions. These intentions may be expressed with increasing variety of words or word combinations as vocabulary increases. The variety of intentions expressed through language also increases. By 4 years of age, children are able to express their intentions in indirect, polite ways. This skill is important for social success. For example, it is more socially acceptable to request that a peer share a new toy by saying, "I like your new car. May I see it?" than by saying "Give me that car."

The rudiments of conversational to-and-fro are present in infancy, as babies respond vocally to their caretakers' utterances. During the preschool years, the length of conversations and degree of topic maintenance is highly dependent on the nature of the topic (high versus low interest to children) and strategies used by the conversational partner (asking questions that obligate a response versus a declarative statement). By school age, children are good conversationalists, maintaining and elaborating familiar topics that others initiate, relating new to old conversational material, and taking turns.

The ability to appreciate the perspective of the conversational partner is critical to appropriate conversational behavior and gradually improves throughout childhood and adolescence. Young children think that others share their knowledge; therefore, they sometimes fail to provide sufficient background information to be accurately understood. For example, young children often neglect to provide the necessary referents for pronouns. By 4 years of age, children clearly show a growing ability to consider their listener's informational needs. For example, they produce simpler sentence structure, different types of verbs, and tend to be more directive when speaking to children younger and less linguistically mature than themselves than when speaking to peers or adults. Recognition and correction of communication breakdowns (misunderstandings) also shows gradual improvement throughout childhood and adolescence. Speakers must constantly assess their partner's comprehension of their messages and, if signs of confusion appear, a hypothesis about the source of confusion and the appropriate repair strategy to employ must be made. For the 3-year-old, repair strategies include repetition of the original utterance, sometimes with clearer articulation, and, occasionally, substituting new words or phrases for those that may have caused the confusion in the first place. By third grade, children are much more adept at determining the necessary revisions that must be made to improve the clarity of their messages and they have an extensive repertoire of revision strategies.

Impaired Language Development

Language development may be delayed or disordered. When delayed, language develops in the normal sequence, but at a slowed rate. Disordered development is characterized by the presence of qualitatively abnormal language behaviors and disruption in the normal pattern of development. Delays that are more severe in some subsystems than in others (heterochrony) may also occur, representing a deviant pattern of development. In this chapter, any abnormality in language development is referred to as "impairment." The cause of impairment may be related to developmental processes or it may result from an acquired neurologic insult or disease.

Developmental language impairment occurs more often in boys than in girls. Although the frank signs of language impairment may diminish or even disappear during the school years, challenging language tasks (e.g., dealing with abstract concepts, integrating text-length information) may pose difficulty for children who had preschool language impairment. As children with early language impairment are at risk for academic and social difficulty, it is important that language problems are identified and treated early in life and these youngsters be followed at appropriate intervals through adolescence.

Developmental language impairment may occur in the absence of abnormality in other domains of development. (See Specific Language Impairment, later.) Language impairment is a frequent concomitant of other developmental disorders, such as hearing impairment, mental retardation, and autism/pervasive developmental disorder. In most cases of developmental disorder involving language impairment, etiology is unknown and no clear neuroanatomic or neurophysiologic basis can be identified.

Language impairment may affect a single language subsystem (e.g., grammatical development) or a combination of language subsystems. The degree to which each subsystem is impaired may also vary. The specific manifestations of language impairment vary from child to child, even within a single developmental disorder (e.g., autism). Thus, a speech-language evaluation is necessary to describe patterns of strength, weakness, and idiosyncracy for each child with language impairment. This said, some general characteristics of language behavior associated with various developmental disorders are described.

Mental Retardation

Children with mental retardation may or may not exhibit language difficulties that are commensurate with the degree of their cognitive impairment. A careful speech-language evaluation is needed to determine if a superimposed language impairment exists. Many individuals with mental retardation exhibit phonological and social language difficulties that are not measurable on intelligence tests or standard language tests. These difficulties may be addressed in intervention programs, decreasing their pejorative influence on the child's social acceptability. Some children with mental retardation with low IQ or poor intelligibility of speech may benefit from augmentative communication systems.

Attention-Deficit Hyperactivity Disorder (ADHD)

Attention-deficit hyperactivity disorder (ADHD) is characterized by difficulties with sustaining attention, impulse control, and overactivity. Although well controlled studies that characterize the nature of communication deficit in ADHD are sparse, professionals and parents often note the coexistence of such problems. Problems with comprehending abstract language relationships (e.g., metaphors, humor), integrating information, producing coherent discourse, word finding, and social language may be seen. Most often noted is social language (pragmatic) impairment. For example, children with ADHD often fail to adequately assess situational cues that are critical for adequately interpreting and formulating social and linguistic aspects of messages. Such cues include facial expressions, body language, and tone of voice. This problem may lead to the production of off-topic responses, seemingly insensitive or rude remarks, and so on. Conversational rules may be broken when children with ADHD are overtalkative or interrupt, failing to respect turn-taking conventions. The ability to organize and monitor information for expression is often impaired in children with ADHD, even those without learning disability (Tannock, Purvis, & Schachar, 1993). Problems with frustration or outbursts of anger may be experienced by children with ADHD and impairments of language expression. The youngsters often do not anticipate the consequences of their behaviors and may not understand why they are rejected by others. Rejection by peers may lead to problems with self-esteem and social isolation, limiting the child's opportunities to learn from unimpaired peer models of social and language behavior.

The communication problems of children with ADHD may not be readily observed in brief, highly structured interviews such as those taking place in a physician's office. Adding to the obscurity of language impairment, early language milestones may have been acquired within an acceptable time frame, grammatical errors may be subtle or absent, and comprehension may seem adequate within the physician's office. Children with ADHD should receive careful speech-language screenings that specifically focus on aspects of language processing and formulation that are not easily observed in casual encounters. Particular scrutiny of word retrieval, story production and comprehension, abstract language, and social language is important in the speech-language evaluation. If direct intervention is not deemed necessary, the speech-language pathologist can help teachers and parents develop appropriate expectations for the child with ADHD, and to develop strategies to facilitate the child's success in learning and social contexts. With appropriate environmental management, substantial reduction in emotional outbursts and self-esteem problems may occur.

Autism

Autism is a neurodevelopmental disorder characterized by language, social, and behavioral abnormalities. All children with autism have abnormalities in language development. Some begin producing a few words at an appropriate age only to stop speaking before 2 years of age, and may or may not acquire a functional verbal communication system at a later age. Others speak, perhaps late, exhibiting atypical language behavior. Others never acquire spoken language, sometimes because of severe speech motor difficulties (e.g., apraxia of speech). If a child with autism is not speaking by 5 years of age, prognosis for spoken language is poor. Nonverbal and verbal children with autism with severe articulation abnormalities should be evaluated for the appropriateness of an augmentative communication system. Such a system may be simple gestures, sign language, photo/picture/symbol communication boards/books, computers, and so on. The efficacy of any system prescribed must be carefully monitored. The system must be employed at home and at school with frequency and consistency to be effective.

Some children with autism are unmotivated to have social engagement or to communicate. Others are very interested in social interaction, but their lack of social insight, communication abnormalities, difficulty taking others' perspectives, poor grasp of social rules and subtle cues, among other deficits, make it difficult for them to interact appropriately. Environmental opportunities to communicate should be clearly structured into the daily routine for children with autism, with verbal and physical modeling and prompting provided when necessary.

Verbal children with autism will vary somewhat in the specific characteristics of their communicative abilities and behavior. Prelanguage vocal and social skills are often impaired (e.g., babbling, vocal turn-taking, gaze patterns, gestural imitation, symbolic gesture, etc.). Nonverbal behaviors are not used appropriately to modulate and augment spoken language. For example, facial expressions, vocal intonation, gaze patterns, and physical distance held between others may be abnormal.

Features of spoken language are also abnormal. Some children with autism frequently repeat part of or entire sentences spoken to them, either immediately or later (echolalia). This repetition may be mixed with words or phrases that the child has self-generated and may or may not be used for communication. Thus, the old view that echolalia is an undesirable behavior that should be extinguished is no longer generally accepted among autism experts (Prizant & Duchan, 1981). A speech-language pathologist may help to determine the degree to which echolalia is present and its use for a particular child.

In general, children with autism have difficulty learning linguistic rules. Their utterances tend to be somewhat stereotyped. This is because they tend to memorize phrases and use them without modification to express a particular meaning, regardless of the social situation. They lack the linguistic flexibility to change the wording to suit the social situation and may not have the perspective-taking ability to determine which changes would make their expression acceptable to the context. Thus, youngsters with autism often produce socially awkward or gauche expressions.

Children with autism have particular difficulty with abstract concepts. Words may be associated with idiosyncratic meanings and therefore used inappropriately, leading to confusion on the part of the listener and misunderstanding for the child with autism when the word is used by others. Thus, figurative language, humor, and words with multiple meanings (e.g., "run") pose problems for the child with autism. Figures of speech such as, "She cried her eyes out," are often interpreted literally and can cause the child to become anxious without the communicative partner recognizing the reason. Such difficulty with abstract language affects academic success and social interactions.

Children with autism have difficulty attending to salient information in their verbal and nonverbal world. They may become preoccupied with small details in a conversation or a part of a toy during play. They also have great difficulty integrating information presented in conversations, stories, television programs, and books. They fail to get the "big picture," leading to difficulty identifying the main point of a television program or of what others say to them. Comprehension of logical relationships is also difficult for children with autism. They require concrete language input, with frequent checks to determine their level of comprehension.

Conversation is often difficult for children with autism, even those who desire social relationships. Their tendency toward concrete interpretations leads to difficulty comprehending indirect speech acts (e.g., saying "Don't you think it's hot in here?" to request that a window be opened). The difficulties discussed above, coupled with preoccupations with specific topics, difficulty maintaining others' topics, tendency to interrupt or engage in a monologue, and problems interpreting subtle social cues make the person with autism a challenging conversational partner.

Some critical components of the educational program for children with autism include: a highly structured routine that is systematically varied, providing the autistic child with a picture or symbol "schedule" so that transitions are better understood and predicted, appropriate reinforcements for successful attention and performance, well-planned interaction with unimpaired peers, programming for generalization of skills developed within one context, reduction of distracting stimuli, language input and opportunities for social use of language that is developmentally appropriate, and educational goals that are designed to meet each child's functional and academic capacities.

Specific Language Impairment

One subgroup of children show language impairment without concurrent deficiency in hearing, vision, IQ, frank neurological signs, obvious sensory or oral motor deficits, or psychiatric disorder. This group has been labeled specifically language-impaired (SLI). Like all other groups of children with language impairment, the SLI group is neither homogeneous in type or severity of disorder. Any or all of the language subsystems may be affected in receptive and/or expressive domains. Children with SLI may exhibit difficulties with attention and impulsivity, adding to their difficulties in conversational situations.

School-aged children with SLI often exhibit deficits that are characteristic of the child with specific learning disabilities, including reading difficulties involving word recognition and text comprehension. In a follow-up study of preschool children with language impairment, Aram and Hall (1989) report that most continued to have language impairment when school-aged. More than half experienced academic difficulties. The literature indicates that the nature of the language impairment may be an important factor in predicting reading disorders in children (Bishop & Adams, 1990). Thus, early speech-language assessments and intervention programs may minimize the risk of reading disability for some children (Catts, 1993).

Grammatical morphemes (e.g., past tense markers such as -*ed*, and so on) present a particular challenge for children with SLI (Leonard, 1989). Research indicates that children with SLI learn grammatical markers in a normal pattern, but at a slower than typical rate (Paul & Alforde, 1993). Although their sentences may be similar in length to those of their peers without impairment, they produce fewer complex grammatical forms than those peers. Ungrammatical sentences are also produced more frequently by youngsters with SLI than normal. Difficulty comprehending complex sentences may affect development in other areas of language development (Leonard, 1989).

Semantic development may also be impaired. Typically, children with SLI exhibit single-word vocabulary comprehension that is superior to their ability to define words or to name words on confrontation. In fact, if we test comprehension of the primary meaning of single words on vocabulary tests such as the *PPVT-R* (Dunn & Dunn, 1981), we will not detect the semantic comprehension problems of children with SLI. School-aged children with SLI often have difficulty comprehending specific categories of words (e.g., spatial, temporal, kinship terms). These problematic words do not refer to isolated objects, actions, or events. Rather, they refer to relationships between objects and/or persons, requiring that the child keep more than one referent in mind. Difficulty retrieving words has been reported in many children with language impairment. Fewer ideas (or semantic relationships) are expressed by children with SLI than unimpaired peers, despite the production of sentences that are equal in length.

Pragmatic skills are sometimes impaired in children with SLI. When present, pragmatic difficulty may be characterized as an impairment in adjusting their message (e.g., clarifying misunderstandings) in response to feedback from the listener and problems adjusting their language and manner of speaking to changes in social context (e.g., authority figures vs. close peers and family, considering background information or language limitations that the listener is likely to have, etc.).

Learning Disability

Many children with specific learning disabilities have concomitant specific speech and/or language difficulties. A growing awareness of the importance of language development for academic success has led to a shift in the use of the label learning disabled. This label is now often applied to preschool children with language impairment who are identified as SLI, because the early language difficulties are viewed as an early manifestation of learning disability. Aram and Nation (1980) report that about 40% of their preschool subjects with language impairment later showed difficulty with mathematics and reading in elementary school.

Many students with learning disabilities develop early speech and language milestones within normal age limits, but exhibit functionally significant language difficulties by third grade. This fact was recently highlighted in a study of students with learning disabilities in reading, written expression, and/or mathematics, but supposedly normal spoken language abilities. These students were found to have impaired narrative discourse (story telling) skills in comparison to nondisabled children (Roth & Spekman, 1986). This study, as well as clinical experience, demonstrates that language functioning is best defined through the speech-language pathologist's administration of standardized and nonstandardized assessment procedures.

Other aspects of language are also impaired in children with learning disabilities. Impaired phonological abilities appear to be the cause of reading disorder in a subgroup of children with learning disabilities (Pennington, 1991). Some have postulated that similar impairments in information processing underlie deficits in spoken (comprehension and expression) and written language (spelling, reading) in these children. Children with learning disabilities also often have impaired metalinguistic ability, resulting in difficulty detecting and revising grammatical errors in sentences, identifying the individual speech sounds that constitute a word, breaking words into syllables, and so on. Related to this impairment is the difficulty some children with learning disabilities have in monitoring their own comprehension of written or spoken information, often not knowing when to request clarification. Other language deficits seen in children with learning disabilities parallel those that characterize children with SLI.

CONCLUSION

Many children with developmental delay will have abnormal communication abilities. As has been pointed out in preceding chapters, deficits in communication abilities typically occur in settings of associated deficits of cognitive, motor, and social-adaptive function. The variability with which speech and language abnormalities may be expressed within and across specific developmental disorders makes individualized assessment and programming a necessity for any child suspected of having communication difficulties. Because communication is so fundamental and impacts many facets of a child's and families' life, early identification leading to early intervention is paramount.

CHAPTER 5

CHILDREN WITH DEVELOPMENTAL DISABILITIES: ANALYSIS AND MODIFICATION OF BEHAVIOR PROBLEMS

Michael F. Cataldo, Ph.D.
Keith J. Slifer, Ph.D.
Jane A. Summers, Ph.D.

Children with developmental disabilities have primary, neurologically based disabling conditions (e.g., mental retardation, cerebral palsy, learning disabilities, attention-deficit hyperactivity disorder (ADHD), and the like). These conditions are indicative of irreversible damage to the central nervous system, are chronic, and can be expected to affect individuals across their lifespan. In contrast, statistics show that children with developmental disabilities have an increased variety of behavioral and emotional problems, these problems are, to a great degree, secondary to (or derivative of) the primary underlying developmental disability. As such, the behavior problems, as opposed to the primary neurologically based disabling condition(s), are mutable. That is, by the careful application of knowledge about learning and behavior, we can maximize the potential of individuals with developmental disabilities despite their underlying neurologically based handicapping condition(s).

Obviously, many factors contribute to the behavior of an individual in any particular situation at any given point in time. Factors especially relevant to children with developmental disabilities include genetic influences, perceptual, motor and cognitive abilities, and medical (e.g., neurological, psychiatric, etc.) status. This chapter discusses an additional set of factors related to learning. These considerations come from an area of psychology called behavioral psychology (also sometimes termed Skinnerian psychology, operant psychology, and behavior analysis). The theoretical basis for behavioral psychology proceeds from the idea that observable behavior and its relationship to environmental events is a particularly useful subject matter on which to base a science of behavior. With this premise, hypothetical constructs about the meaning of behavior, what a child is thinking or feeling, and internal structures or states are avoided, because such constructs are considered unnecessary rather than unreal.

A most useful finding from research in behavioral psychology is that behavior is partially a function of its consequences. That is, in addition to all the other factors that determine how a child behaves, the consequences of a child's behavior greatly affects how the child behaves in the future. The infant may cry because of a genetic predisposition to do so, especially when motivated by hunger, pain, or some other discomfort. But the parent's response to such vocalization teaches that the infant's behavior has the function of producing a result from the parent. Thus, what may initially occur as a reflex response can quickly also become a learned, or operant, behavior. Operant learning occurs in the first few days of life and we suspect has great survival value.

The child with developmental disabilities and a severe communication disorder will have the same (or perhaps greater) need to communicate as the normal child. Such a child can be expected to explore his or her behavior and its effect on the environment until consequences demonstrate which behaviors can be relied on to gain attention, assistance, specific items, such as favorite toys, preferred food, relief from physical discomfort, avoidance of unwanted situations, and so on. That such learned behavior takes the form of screaming, tantrums, self-injury, aggression, smiling, pointing, leading a parent to an object rather than saying "please come here," "help me," "more," "dollie," "juice," or "no," does not make the behavior any less functional or adaptive to the individual child, just nontypical, nonnormal, and problematic to the parent and professional.

Problem behaviors are more likely to occur in children who have medical and neurological conditions, be they acute or chronic in nature. For example, in the general population the frequency of behavior problems is estimated to be 5–15%. The frequency doubles for those with chronic physical disease and further increases when multiple handicaps exist (Haggerty, 1986). For individuals with mental retardation, behavioral dependency and significant problematic behavior increases with the degree of mental impairment. The incidence of severe aggression, self-injury and property destruction is as low as 2% for the mild range of retardation and as high as 17% for the profound range (Schroeder, Rojahn, & Oldenquist, 1991). Further, for the severest form of behavior problems, the cost to society is considerable in that severe self-injury and aggression are estimated to involve 20,000 to 25,000 individuals at a direct care cost exceeding $3 billion per year (National Institutes of Health [NIH], 1991).

Learning is a cumulative process. That is, continued association between a behavior and particular consequences greatly strengthens the likelihood that behavior will be used to obtain those consequences in the future. This learning history not only predisposes certain behaviors to occur in the future but explains their continued occurrence. A child may cry and scream because of anger or frustration. (Laboratory animals, when experimentally "frustrated," become aggressive.) The parent's response to crying and screaming can teach the child that this behavior can produce attention, comforting acts from the parent (such as hugging, kissing, presentation of preferred objects) and a change in the current situation. Even anger on the parents' part could strengthen a child's crying behavior, if gaining the parents' attention (regardless of the form) is what is sought. Thus, a child who is angry and frustrated at bedtime when the TV is turned off may cry and scream. If this produces an extra hour of TV, bed time snacks, long discussion from the parent, and the like, then crying and screaming (e.g., tantrums) will over time come to have an established learning history and will continue to be used by the child even if not always producing the desired consequence. Thus, a behavior may initially occur for a variety of reasons, but how the child's environment responds to the behavior determines how it is elaborated and maintained in the future.

So well studied and consistent is this "behavior-consequence" relationship throughout the phylogenetic scale that we often consider it a basic and necessary adaptation strategy of organisms. As genetics represents a strategy for adaptation within a species across generations, learning represents a strategy for adaptation within an individual across a lifetime. To the extent that this is true, the "behavior-consequence" relation can be a powerful tool in changing behavior regardless of (or despite) additional factors influencing its existence (e.g., genetics, cognitive level, etc.).

With this introduction, the remainder of this chapter will outline the *basic tenets*, concepts in behavioral psychology on which clinical applications are based, and then provide examples of how behavioral psychology has been used with *typical problems* of children with developmental disabilities and in the special case of *autism*.

THE BASICS OF A BEHAVIOR ANALYTIC APPROACH TO BEHAVIOR PROBLEMS

Over the past 25 years the field of behavioral psychology has developed an extensive literature on the assessment and treatment of maladaptive behavior and the establishment of daily living skills in individuals with developmental disabilities. The methodology and procedures developed within this field have allowed such individuals increased opportunity for participation in the mainstream of community, school, and workplace settings.

Although the behavior and learning difficulties of persons with developmental disabilities are neurologically based, research in behavioral psychology has resulted in a systematic and powerful approach for both increasing and decreasing specific behaviors despite cognitive limitations, learning disabilities, and collateral aberrant behavior. Central to this approach is the use of three terms that describe the contingent relationship between behavior and environmental events or stimuli. These three terms are: *antecedents, behavior, and consequences.* Any behavior analysis, regardless of the presenting problem or symptoms, must consider these components. First, the symptom or behavior of interest must be described or operationalized in sufficient detail to be reliably measured by direct observation or mechanical means. Second, an attempt to understand the variables causing or maintaining the occurrence of a targeted behavior is initiated by observing temporal relationships among events in the physical, social, and biological environment in relation to target behavior. Thus, events that reliably precede the behavior (antecedents) and those that reliably follow it (consequences) are selected for experimental manipulation. By objectively measuring the behavior while manipulating these temporally related events, it is possible to demonstrate manipulations that alter the frequency of the behavior. This behavior analysis forms the process by which often powerful interventions have been developed for a variety of behavior problems encountered in children, including those with developmental disabilities.

The simplest and some of the most dramatic treatment techniques have come from differentially arranging consequences so as to increase or decrease desired or undesired behaviors, respectively. These basic behavior analytic techniques have been extended and refined to study the motivation or "reasons" why certain seemingly maladaptive behaviors persist. This extension of behavior analysis has been termed *functional analysis* because behavior persists (theory holds) because of its function. During a functional analysis, a variety of brief antecedent-behavior-consequence situations are arranged and the rates of behavior in each type of situation are noted. By comparing rates, assumptions can be made about which consequences maintain high rates of behavior. The importance of this functional analysis approach is that it permits empirically based behavioral diagnosis for behavior problems, allowing the most parsimonious and efficacious treatment course to be selected.

A further extension of early behavior analytic work has been the study of relationships between groups of behaviors. The notion here is that behaviors that result in similar consequences (i.e., have similar function) can become related to each other and form response classes. A response class would then have many of the same properties of a discrete behavior. The importance of this response class approach is that by properly arranging learning conditions, one can change an entire class of behaviors by providing differential consequences for only a few of the behaviors in the response class.

Each of these behavior analytic approaches are explained with specific examples in the next section. As complicated as they may sound, each can be translated into practical programs for staff, teachers, and parents. A key to this "translation" is the use of objective measures of behavior, usually accomplished by noting or counting the behavior for a period of time before and during the treatment phases. Charting or graphing these behavioral data becomes the behavioral equivalent of blood and urine analyses, radiological imaging, cognitive and neurological testing, and the like, in that these behavioral data provide similar objective determination on the status of the target problem over time and across treatment efforts. The two most common behavior analytic approaches are to note and display behavioral data across sequences of no treatment versus treatment (reversal method) or sequentially across behaviors or settings, and the like (multiple baseline method).

It will be very useful for the reader to become familiar with the basic methods by which behavioral psychologists display and make judgements about behavior change. Points made later in this chapter are illustrated by data from studies in behavioral psychology, and familiarity with methods for graphing data will make it easier to understand these points. Also, in treatment situations, graphic displays of a child's behavior and a child's progress through treatment applications are shared with parents and teachers so that all may become involved in the decision process for treatment. Therefore, by way of introduction, Figures 5–1, 5–2a, and 5–2b provide typical examples of the ways in which behavioral data are arranged in making decisions. These graphs are from actual studies reported in the research literature.

The first method shown is in Figure 5–1 and uses a technique of obtaining baseline data, applying a treatment technique, then removing the treatment technique, and finally initiating the treatment again (i.e., reversal method or design). The data shown in Figure 5–1 demonstrate this technique and are from a study investigating the effects of nonverbal teacher approval on the attending behavior of students in a classroom. During the baseline condition (labeled as A) students were attentive in the classroom about 50% of the time (ranging from approximately 45 to 60%). When a teacher's nonverbal attention or approval was made contingent on children's attending, the childrens' behavior increased to approximately 80% (ranging from 65 to 85%). To test the likelihood that this increase was indeed caused by the change in the teacher's behavior, a brief reversal was instituted back to the baseline condition. The subsequent decrease in the childrens' attending behavior increases our confidence that the changes noted were due to nonverbal teacher approval. This confidence level goes up even further

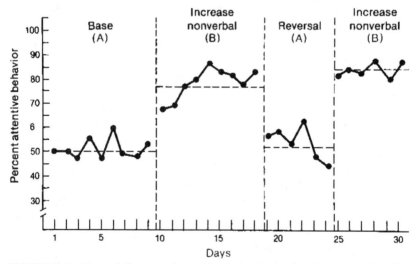

FIGURE 5–1. Mean daily rate of attentive behavior in the class. *From* Kazdin, A. E., & Klock, J. (1973). The effect of nonverbal teacher approval on student attentive behavior. *Journal of Applied Behavior Analysis, 6,* 643–654. Reprinted by permission.

when the treatment condition of increased nonverbal teacher approval was reinstituted a final time on days 25 through 31.

Another method for displaying behavior data and testing treatment interventions is called a multiple baseline design. In this technique (shown in Figures 5–2a and 5–2b), baselines are collected on a behavior in a variety of situations such as shown in Figure 5–2a, or on a variety of behaviors such as shown in Figure 5–2b, or across any other measure or dependent variable of interest. In the multiple baseline technique, an intervention is applied at different points in time and the resulting changes in behavior over baseline levels are used to determine the confidence that one has in the effectiveness of the treatment. Thus, in the case of the behavior shown in Figure 5–2a, a behavior modification technique of ignoring "bizarre responses" in a summer camp situation was attempted across camp settings of "walking on a trail," "in the dining hall," "in the cabins," and "in an educational setting." The dramatic changes in the childrens' responses between baseline and this intervention technique, particularly in the walk on trail and dining hall activities, indicates that this approach may have had some effect on behavior. Further, that the behavior only changed when the treatment technique was instituted, even though it was instituted at different points in time, greatly increases our confidence that the changes were from the intervention as stated. Similarly, in Figure 5–2b, by instituting social skills training at three different points in time across four behaviors, the changes in behavior for the first three behaviors shown increase our confidence that this type of training was indeed effective for at least those first three behaviors.

APPLICATIONS TO TYPICAL BEHAVIOR PROBLEMS

The analytic approach of considering behavior in terms of antecedents, behavior, and consequences, and the use of graphic treatment designs as described has been applied successfully to the remediation of a wide variety of behavior problems. The goals of these applications have been to either decrease unwanted behaviors or increase those that will benefit the individual by increasing his or her independence and integration into more normalized settings. Examples of applications to decrease behavior include programs to reduce or eliminate self-injurious and stereotyped behavior, aggression and destructive behavior. Areas where behaviors have been established and increased include self-help skills such as feeding, independent toileting, toothbrushing, and menstrual hygiene; language and social behavior, such as social greetings, nonvocal communication skills, naming of objects, and augmented communication;

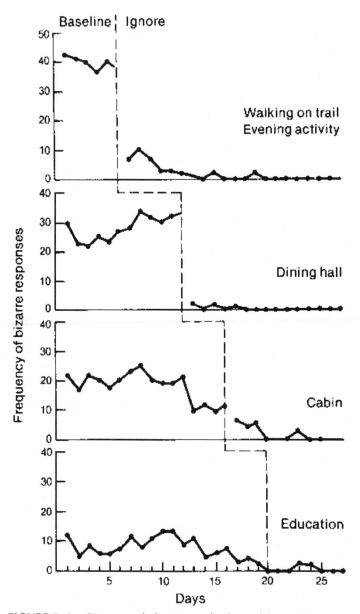

FIGURE 5–2a. Bizarre verbalizations of a brain-damaged boy at summer camp. Baseline—before the intervention. Ignore—turning away from the boy for bizarre verbalizations; attending to appropriate verbalizations. *From* Allen, G. J. (1973). Case study: Implementation of behavior modification techniques in summer camp settings. *Behavior Therapy, 4,* 570–75. Reprinted by permission.

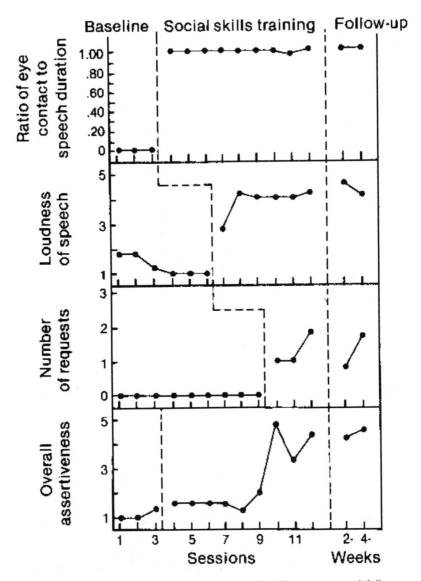

FIGURE 5-2b. Sessions during baseline, social skills training, and follow-up for Jane. *From* Bornstein, M. R., Bellack, A. S., & Hersen, M. (1977). Social-skills training for unassertive children: A multiple-baseline analysis. *Journal of Applied Behavior Analysis, 10,* 183-195. Reprinted by permission.

vocational skills, such as janitorial tasks, job skills, and workshop tasks; community survival skills, such as crossing the street, leisure activities, clothing selection, laundry, eating in public places, and purchasing items in a store. A few examples of specific programs will demonstrate how the basic analytic techniques described above are used in practical applications.

One of the best known studies in the field demonstrated methods for rapidly toilet-training (both bladder and bowel) individuals with profound mental handicaps and up to 45 years of institutional incontinence (Azrin & Foxx, 1971). Nine profoundly retarded adults underwent brief but intensive behavioral training (median of 4 days). This required a combination of antecedent changes in the physical environment as well as arranging consistent differential consequences for successful use of the toilet and soiling accidents. The participants were given frequent fluids to drink, thereby increasing opportunities for voiding and they were prompted to sit on the toilet at half-hour intervals. Edible reinforcers and social praise were provided, contingent on approximations of undressing and dressing for toilet use, for sitting on the toilet, and for successful elimination in the toilet. When accidents occurred, the participants were required to participate in a cleanliness training routine in which they obtained fresh clothing from the laundry, undressed, received a shower, dressed, hand washed the soiled clothes, and cleaned the soiled area on the chair or floor.

The participants also were provided with two types of apparatus to facilitate learning. The first was special training pants equipped with a device that detected moisture from urine or feces and immediately sounded a signal—an electronic tone. This helped both participants and staff to know immediately when an accident had occurred. The second apparatus was similar, involving a plastic bowl with moisture detector that was inserted into the toilet and signaled the occurrence of successful toilet use. Using this combination of techniques, incontinence was reduced immediately by about 90% and eventually decreased to near-zero. The staff effort, after the initial training, was reduced considerably. Maintenance involved conducting periodic cleanliness checks, intermittently reinforcing continence and toilet use (with praise and scheduled snacks), and prompting cleanliness training on the few occasions when an accident occurred. Thus, by conceptualizing continence as a complex and lengthy chain of responses in relation to social, environmental and physiological stimuli, which could be analyzed and altered using operant conditioning (planned consequences), daytime accidents were virtually eliminated in these participants with profound disabilities. The procedures in this study have been varied, elaborated, and consistently replicated with adults and children across the developmental spectrum. In the past decade, behavior analytic approaches using a simple antecedent-behavior-consequence viewpoint have shown how even children with disabilities such as spina bifida, in which continence was previously thought to be neurologically impossible, have attained at least partial continence (Whitehead, Parker, Masek, Cataldo, & Freeman, 1981).

The literature now describes hundreds of studies on the pivotal role of behavioral approaches in helping individuals with primary neurologically based disabilities obtain skills that afford them greater independence and human dignity in their home environment. For example, behaviors can be taught that allow persons with mental retardation to participate more safely and freely within the community (Page, Iwata, & Neef, 1976). In this study, five students at a center for those with multiple disabilities were taught five specific skills involved in safe street crossing. First, using a classroom model and then conducting sessions in the community, the participants were taught to recognize intersections and to respond correctly to pedestrian signal lights, traffic lights, and stop signs. With the classroom model and a doll to role-play walking through simulated traffic conditions, the participants were taught to make correct responses using contingent praise for appropriate responding. Corrective verbal feedback and demonstrations were provided contingent on errors (dangerous responses). Periodic supervised trials at actual intersections in the community were used to demonstrate that these skills were actually employed in live traffic situations. In this case, only social consequences were necessary to teach participants not to walk into the street without waiting for a safe signal and looking left and right for oncoming traffic. These types of adaptive community skills can be taught using basic behavioral methods. They are critical to community placement, successful employment, and greater access to educational and recreational resources for the mentally retarded.

A final example of the traditional antecedent-behavior-consequence approach involves prevention of further neurological impairment. Finney, Russo, and Cataldo (1982) conducted a study demonstrating teaching techniques that are effective in decreasing to very low levels, ingestion of inedible materials (pica) in toddlers and preschool children hospitalized for treatment of lead poisoning. In these children, their pica was thought to be the primary source of lead absorption because of the presence of deteriorating lead-based paint in their homes, producing chips and dust ingested via pica. In these children, developmentally normative oral exploration can result in irreversible cognitive deterioration. Furthermore, the resulting developmental delay may prolong the stage of primarily oral exploration. Without behavioral intervention to reduce the pica, a circular pattern of pica, lead poisoning, cognitive impairment, and continued pica can ensue.

In this study, an initial baseline phase was carried out during which pica behavior was assessed across repeated sessions in a clinical environment. The clinic environment had a variety of items that the children could mouth, but were not dangerous. For example, lead paint chips were simulated by a mixture of water and flour, all items were cleaned thoroughly before being placed in the room, no hard items were small enough to cause a child to be able to swallow them and choke. As shown in Figure 5–3, childrens' pica behavior was quite variable during this baseline phase, ranging from 0 to 100% of intervals observed, and, in fact, appeared to increase over time for at least two of the children (Pam and Nancy). This baseline phase was followed by an intervention sequence that first taught children via differential presentation of praise and snacks to identify edible and inedible objects in the environment. This first intervention phase was called "discrimination

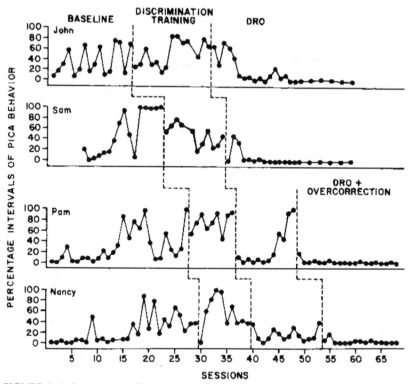

FIGURE 5–3. Percentage of intervals in which pica behavior was observed across experimental conditions for the four subjects. *From* Finney, J. W., Russo, D. C., & Cataldo, M. F. (1982). Reduction of pica in young children with lead poisoning., *Journal of Pediatric Psychology, 7*(2), 197–207. Reprinted by permission.

training" and, as can be seen in Figure 5–3, did not have a consistent impact on pica behavior, although Sam's pica behavior appeared to have decreased somewhat during the discrimination training phase. Next, each child entered a phase of treatment called "DRO," in which differential reinforcement in the form of praise and preferred snacks was arranged contingent upon refraining from pica for increasing intervals. (DRO is a contraction for a procedure called "*d*ifferential *r*einforcement of *0* rate behavior.")

For all three children, this DRO procedure decreased pica behavior. For two of the children, John and Sam, this decrease was sustained for the remainder of the study. Whereas, in Nancy's case, although the pica behavior level was decreased, it was not considered to reach safe levels, and for Pam, pica behavior soon increased to baseline levels. Thus, for the two children who did not have sustained, safe decreases in pica behavior (Pam and Nancy), an additional procedure was added, called "overcorrection." The overcorrection procedure was one in which the child's mouth and teeth were brushed with a toothbrush and mouthwash each time pica behavior occurred. As can be seen in Figure 5–3, the combination of DRO and overcorrection for Pam and Nancy consistently reduced pica behavior to safe levels.

Thus, in all cases, simply teaching the child to discriminate edible from inedible materials did not significantly decrease the frequency of their pica. In two cases, differentially reinforcing the absence of pica resulted in near elimination of this dangerous oral behavior. The other two cases required the contingent oral hygiene procedure (overcorrection), in addition to differential reinforcement of other behavior to adequately suppress pica.

This study demonstrates how the objective measurement of target problem behavior and a systematic approach using single-subject experimental research methodology can illuminate effective intervention approaches to health threatening behavior. Behavioral interventions can make an important contribution to the well-being of children who have neurological disorders or are at risk of acquired neurological damage as a result of the interaction between their behavior and variables in their environment.

FUNCTIONAL ANALYSIS

As mentioned in the previous section, these basic behavioral methods have been extended to consider a more sophisticated set of issues. This recent line of work attempts to identify environmental conditions that serve to promote and maintain behavior problems and to teach more appropriate strategies for communication, interaction, and adaptation. Over a number of years, the motivation, or "reasons," for behavior problems in children with severe disabilities, many of whom have a variety of diagnoses, have been delineated as: (1) the individual's desire to escape or avoid certain people, situations, or events; (2) a means for the individual to gain access to something, whether tangible (e.g., food, toys) or intangible (social attention); and (3) for self-stimulatory (nonsocial) purposes. As such an analytic approach attempts to determine the function of the behavior, it has been termed a functional analysis approach.

A functional analysis approach to the assessment and treatment of behavior problems involves careful controlled observation. Initially, emphasis is placed on defining or operationalizing the behavior to be observed and measured. Next, quantitative data are gathered, which may include measures of frequency, duration, or intensity. Particular attention is paid to environmental events and factors that may be influencing the behavior, such as the presence or absence of particular persons, changes in schedules or routines, presentation of different tasks or instructional material, and so on. Variables that are presumed to maintain the behavior are manipulated directly and the subsequent effects on children's responding are measured and evaluated. Once the presumed maintaining conditions have been identified, this information is used to formulate a treatment approach that incorporates dual objectives of reducing the problem behavior and providing alternative, socially acceptable strategies that may be used in its place.

For example, a child may bite her arm when she is told to put the toys away. The starting point for a functional analysis involves defining the aberrant behavior(s) in precise terms to facilitate accurate observation and measurement. In this particular example, self-injury may be defined as contact between the teeth and any part of the wrist or forearm.

The next step in the analysis involves observation and data recording. Measurements are taken on the frequency, duration, and intensity of the behavior across a variety of circumstances. A more fine-grained analysis of situational variables may be conducted in order to pinpoint specific factors that may be influencing the behavior. This type of assessment may yield the finding that the behavior occurs only when the child is asked to put away a favorite toy (such as blocks) as opposed to different types of material. The antecedent or trigger for the self-injury may be identified as the teacher's request to the child to put the blocks away and the outcome may be that the teacher allows the child to continue the activity when she engages in the behavior. The assumption is made that the child's self-injury is being used to prolong a favored activity by avoiding or escaping the teacher's request to put the blocks away.

This hypothesis may be tested directly by altering the events surrounding the behavior. For instance, the teacher may be instructed under different conditions to: (1) allow the child to continue to play with the blocks after the self-injury occurs; (2) tell the child to stop biting her arm because she may hurt herself; or (3) ignore the self-injury and remove the blocks. Multiple observations are conducted under different conditions to establish differential rates of responding and to evaluate the validity of the hypothesis that the behavior serves as a means to avoid the teacher's request. If this is the case and biting is not causing tissue damage, then the child should bite her arm more frequently if she is allowed to continue playing with the blocks after engaging in self-injury than when she is ignored and the blocks are put away.

The assessment process is closely linked with the development of treatment strategies. In the case where the self-injury is used as an avoidance strategy, the approach may be to prompt or assist the child to put the blocks away and to not provide any social attention (e.g., a verbal reprimand) for the behavior. Reductions in self-injury should occur over time, because the behavior is no longer being reinforced by allowing the child to continue with the activity. A second component to a treatment strategy involves teaching the child a new response that can be used to replace the aberrant behavior. For instance, the child may be trained to request "More time please" as a more appropriate way to prolong the activity. Hence, the link between the aberrant behavior and the expected or desired consequences is broken or uncoupled and a new association is formed in its place.

Hypothetical data are presented in Figure 5–4, depicting the occurrence of self-injury as a function of attention and escape-related variables. During the assessment phase, data on the rates of self-injury were collected under the following conditions: (1) escape from demands, when the child was allowed to continue playing with the blocks after engaging in self-injury; (2) social attention, when the teacher provided a verbal reprimand following the occurrence of the behavior ("Stop, you'll hurt yourself"); and (3) no attention or escape from demands, when social attention was withdrawn after the behavior occurred and the child was prompted to comply with the request to put the blocks away. Rates of self-injury were highest under the escape from demands condition, at intermediate levels during the social attention condition, and lowest during the no attention or escape from demands condition. Data were replicated across conditions to establish and evaluate differential rates of responding. A treatment program was implemented once a clear and consistent pattern was identified. Treatment consisted of

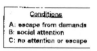

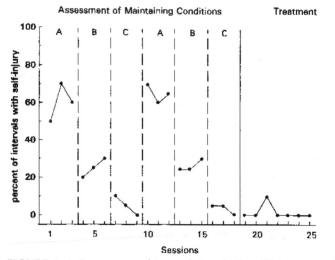

FIGURE 5–4. Percentage of intervals in which self-injury was observed across assessment and treatment conditions. *From* hypothetical data.

several components: (1) withdrawing social attention for the self-injury; (2) prompting compliance with the teacher's request to put the blocks away; and (3) training a verbal response to request more time to play. These data indicate that the treatment approach was successful in eliminating the child's self-injury in this setting.

An early example (Carr & Durand, 1985a, 1985b) of the usefulness and elegance of a functional analysis method demonstrated that systematic analysis of the environmental conditions under which a disruptive behavior occurs can result in a better appreciation of the variables maintaining the behavior and can guide in the selection and teaching of safer and more socially appropriate responses to fulfill the same purpose. The data showed that behavior problems (including aggression, tantrums, and self-injury) displayed by four developmentally disabled children were most likely to occur in situations in which there was a low level of adult attention or a high level of task difficulty, and when children were taught to verbally request attention, assistance with tasks or both, behavior problems reliably decreased. In this study, rather simple techniques such as verbal prompting and response contingent affection and praise were used to teach the children to make simple verbal responses ("Am I doing good work?", "I don't understand") in situations where they presumably used disruptive behavior to functionally communicate the same thing. The reasons that a child learns to use disruptive behavior for communication continue to be debated in the field, but it is widely accepted that this occurs, at least in part, because neurologically based disabilities make language more taxing than other motor and vocal responses.

RESPONSE CLASSES

In addition to a functional analysis, recent elaboration of behavior analytic techniques have involved the study and clinical application of relationships between behaviors. As mentioned previously, classes of behavior could be changed by providing differential consequences for only a few members of a class. So for example, following a parent's instructions (a behavior critical to development and safety of young children and those with lower levels of cognitive functioning) could be increased greatly for all instructions by training and reinforcing only a handful of instructions.

Equally intriguing is the use of this response class notion when groups of behaviors vary inversely with each other. That is, for example, when a group of behaviors "A" increase, another group "B" decreases. In this situation providing differential positive consequences for group "A" would increase "A" and also decrease "B," even though no direct intervention was carried out for "B." When group "B" is maladaptive and inappropriate or dangerous behavior, this response class approach would permit the reduction of problem behaviors by a totally positive approach based on reinforcing other behaviors.

Thus, analysis of response relationships offers the potential for designing treatment procedures that are more economical and entail less risk for misuse than many we currently employ. This is demonstrated by the study of the relationship between compliance and correlated problem behaviors of young children with developmental disabilities (Cataldo, Ward, Russo, Riordan, & Bennett, 1986). The children were presented with a variety of motor problems, including destructive behavior. The effect of providing positive reinforcement for cooperation with adult requests was looked at using a multiple baseline approach wherein three conditions were compared, no reinforcement, reinforcement contingent on the passage of time but not behavior, and reinforcement contingent on cooperation or compliance.

The data are displayed in Figure 5–5 and show that: (1) compliance covaries with problem behaviors; (2) sustained covariation occurred

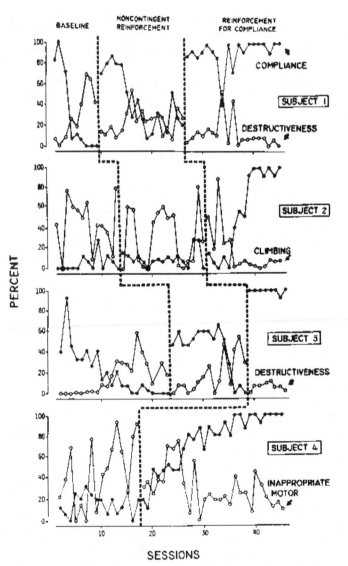

FIGURE 5–5. The percentage of compliance with instructions (closed circles) and percent occurrence of a problem behavior (open circles) across subjects and experimental conditions. *From* Cataldo, M. F., Ward, E. M., Russo, D. C., Riordan, M., & Bennett, D. (1986). Compliance and correlated problem behavior in children: Effects of contingent and noncontingent reinforcement. *Analysis and Intervention in Developmental Disabilities, 6,* 265–282. Reprinted by permission.

only when reinforcement was contingent on compliance; (3) substantially large but transient increases in compliance and decreases in problem behavior during noncontingent reinforcement occurred for those children who initially demonstrated high compliance and low levels of aberrant behavior during baseline. Thus, both Subject 1 and Subject 2 had initial high rates of compliance during baseline that were not maintained during that condition or during the following condition, noncontingent reinforcement. Whereas the data for Subject 1 and Subject 3 were different from those of Subject 2 and 4 during the first two conditions, all four children demonstrated high rates of compliance and low levels of destructiveness when parents praised and otherwise reinforced cooperation. These results suggest that treatment procedures based on response relationship strategies can be used to provide solely positive approaches to increase desired behavior and decrease undesired behavior and that this can be done within a very simple parenting situation.

A similar study by Slifer, Ivancic, Parrish, Page, and Burgio (1986) serves to illustrate the impact of systematic behavior management procedures on the highly disruptive behavior of a profoundly retarded, multiply disabled adolescent. This 13-year-old male was ambulatory, but dependent for all activities of daily living. He was congenitally blind and had no expressive language. His severe aggression, destructiveness, and noncompliance had resulted in expulsion from his special education school, thereby precluding educational opportunities. His aggression included hitting, kicking, biting, grabbing, pinching, and hair pulling. He also hit and bit himself, screamed and threw or broke objects, such as toys. A systematic behavioral assessment showed that his compliance with adult instructions was very inconsistent and often quite low, particularly with family members. Aggression in response to adult instructions was typical and frequent.

Figure 5–6 displays data on his compliance and aggression. Behavioral treatment for this adolescent consisted of: (1) providing positive reinforcement (praise, affection, edibles) contingent on compliance with adult instructions, (2) manual guidance to perform a requested task contingent on noncompliance, and (3) never terminating demands contingent on aggression. With these procedures, the child's behavior was quickly brought under instructional control. Compliance increased substantially. Aggression and other disruptive behavior also decreased significantly, despite the absence of any direct consequence for their occurrence. Figure 5–6 shows these improvements across both hospital staff and family members, who were trained to implement the same procedures.

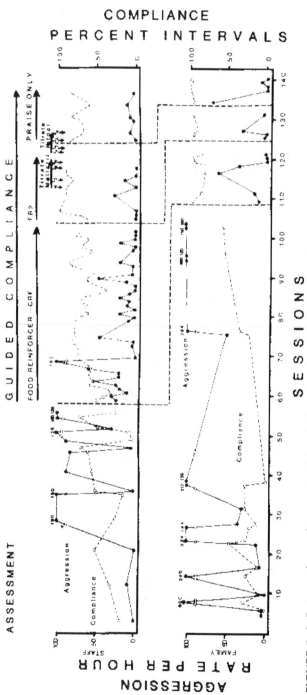

FIGURE 5-6. Rate per hour of aggression (closed circles) and percentage of trials of compliance (open circles) across staff- and family-conducted sessions during assessment, behavioral treatment and withdrawal of neuroleptic medication. *From* Slifer, K. J., Ivancic, M. T., Parrish, J. M., Page, T. J., & Burgio, L. D. (1986). Assessment and treatment of multiple behavior problems exhibited by a profoundly retarded adolescent. *Journal of Behavior Therapy and Experimental Psychiatry, 17*(3), 203–213. Reprinted by permission.

140

CHILDREN WITH AUTISM AND PERVASIVE DEVELOPMENTAL DISORDERS

A recurrent theme of this text is that children with neurodevelopmental delay often manifest an array of problems that arise in response to a primary handicapping condition, such as mental retardation, learning disabilities, language disorders, and so on. In many cases, these problems are reactive in nature and are related to issues concerning adjustment and adaptation to the individual's disability or disorder. Low self-image, negative self-attributions, social withdrawal, aggression, and acting out, among others, may develop if the child becomes a target for ridicule by peers or is confronted by situations in which expectations for their behavior and academic performance are unrealistic or inappropriate.

The task of delineating primary and secondary behavior problems in children with autism and pervasive developmental disorder is more complicated. Autism is characterized by qualitative impairments in communication, socialization, and responsiveness to the environment (American Psychiatric Association, 1987). The severe and chronic nature of the disorder may be attributed to the early and continued involvement of multiple, related psychological systems or areas of functioning; hence, the term "pervasive developmental disorder" (American Psychiatric Association, 1987). Autism is a subtype of pervasive developmental disorder, and may be distinguished from the latter on the basis of the severity and prototypicality of presenting symptoms. The boundaries between autism, pervasive developmental disorder (PDD), global developmental delay, and specific language disorders, however, are often unclear or imprecise (Goodman, 1989; Rutter & Schopler, 1987). For instance, autism is frequently, though not exclusively, associated with mental retardation (Bartak & Rutter, 1976; Rutter & Lockyer, 1967; Wing, 1981). Behavior problems that may be considered as an indication of emotional dysfunction in other groups of children (e.g., social withdrawal, inappropriate affect, lack of empathy for others) are part of the core disturbance in autism. For the remainder of this section, children with markedly deviant communication and interpersonal skills as well as restricted and stereotyped interests will be referred to as autistic, although the disorder may be conceptualized as falling within a broader spectrum, rather than existing as a distinct or separate entity (e.g., Allen, 1988).

Children with autism are generally aberrant in their responding to people and social stimuli. Often, their speech is not used for "social" or interactive purposes (Wing & Attwood, 1987); instead, it is used for the satisfaction of basic physical needs (rather than psychological needs) or is produced in a ritualistic and perseverative manner. Autistic children also have great difficulty understanding or inferring people's thoughts, intentions, and beliefs (Baron-Cohen, 1988; Frith, 1989), as well as the so-called "unwritten" rules for social interactions (Rumsey, 1985). In view of the complex array of skills and disabilities that characterize children's functioning in cognitive, linguistic, and social domains, it is unlikely that the disorder can be attributed to a unitary cause or deficit (Goodman, 1989).

A variety of modalities have been used to try to treat children with autism. Medical intervention has consisted primarily of psychopharmacological approaches. Although the aim of treatment is toward alleviating symptomatology, therapeutic benefits are often far outweighed by the risks and negative side-effects of medication (Sloman, 1991). Psychotherapy and insight-oriented approaches are generally not viable options in view of the individual's impairments in verbal communication and social understanding. Behavior therapy, by contrast, has resulted in demonstrable, stable, and widespread improvements in children's functioning. The next section deals with issues underlying the application of behavioral principles to treating and understanding children with autism.

Learning Characteristics of Children With Autism

Investigators have delineated a number of learning characteristics of children with autism that often pose challenges to intervention. One key characteristic discussed in greater detail pertains to children's attention and responsiveness to the environment.

Overselective Responding

From reviewing the case histories of children with autism, it is apparent that many of these children have appeared unresponsive or totally oblivious to various aspects of their environment from a very early stage in life (Kanner, 1943). Parents often suspected that their children were blind or deaf—so severe was their lack of responsiveness to visual and auditory stimulation (Kanner, 1943; Koegel & Schreibman, 1976; Rutter & Lockyer, 1967). Paradoxically, these same children would concurrently demonstrate a selective awareness of certain environmental features or events (Schreibman & Lovaas, 1973).

Over the past two decades, evidence regarding the selective quality or nature of attention of children with autism has been gathered directly through controlled experimentation, as well as indirectly in an anecdotal manner. The terms "overselective attention" and "stimulus overselectivity" have been used to describe and explain the nature of responding to environmental stimuli by children with autism (Lovaas, Schreibman, Koegel, & Rehm, 1971; Schreibman & Lovaas, 1973; Wilhelm & Lovaas, 1976). Although there is conflicting evidence on the specificity and generalizability of these findings (Gersten, 1980, 1983), many children with autism show evidence of "overselectivity" by attending to restricted or even irrelevant environmental cues (Kolko, Anderson, & Campbell, 1980; Lovaas et al., 1971).

Specialized methodologies have been developed for addressing the problem of overselective attention in children with autism. One area of research deals with attempts to remediate their difficulties. In conditional discrimination training, for example, children are first trained to respond to separate learning features or cues, then later to combinations of these cues (Koegel & Schreibman, 1977; Schreibman, Charlop, & Koegel, 1982). In some studies, orienting tasks or processing instructions have been used to direct the children's attention to various aspects of the training stimuli (e.g., Koegel, Dunlap, Richman, & Dyer, 1981). By contrast, alternative approaches have been used to manage overselective attention by using prompts or guides that emphasize salient or relevant learning cues (Rincover, 1978; Rincover & Ducharme, 1987; Summers, Rincover, & Feldman, 1993).

Behavioral Characteristics of Children With Autism

Behavior problems almost invariably accompany a diagnosis of autism. Although the expression of these problems depends on the individual's age, level of functioning, medical status, severity of autistic symptomatology, and treatment history, behavioral concerns are evident across the full spectrum of the disorder (Minshew & Payton, 1988). Core deficits in communication and socialization often coexist with secondary problems in the form of self-injury, aggression, and tantrums. Lack of social motivation and selective responding to aspects of the environment are also characteristic of these children. These behaviors may stigmatize children, heightening their social withdrawal and isolation, and interfere with or impede their learning and acquisition of new skills.

In the past, many behaviors that are exhibited by children with autism (e.g., echolalia, self-stimulation) were characterized as bizarre, psychotic, or nonfunctional in nature. This notion may have stemmed from the belief that children's behavior was not linked to contextual events and occurred in an unpredictable or random fashion. Examples of this might be the child who tells himself to stop throwing the chair when he becomes upset or agitated, the child who bites her arm when she is told to put the toys away, or the child who stares at lights and flaps his hands for hours. This view has been subsequently modified, in light of extensive evidence that children's behavior is shaped and maintained by environmental factors. Using behaviorally oriented approaches, researchers have identified environmental conditions that maintain these behaviors and use this information as a basis for teaching alternative, more socially acceptable forms of behavior.

Functional Basis for Problem Behaviors

One of the most important advances toward understanding and treating children with autism is the view that their aberrant or inappropriate behaviors serve a communicative function. In children with autism, language deficits are not confined solely to verbal modes of communication. These children also manifest difficulties with nonverbal forms of communication, such as imitating and responding to gestures, interpreting emotions, and so on (Bartak, Rutter, & Cox, 1975; Ricks & Wing, 1975; Wing, 1981; Wing & Attwood, 1987). Children's cognitive and language-based disabilities interact with their social skills deficits, setting the occasion for behavior problems to develop and subsequently be shaped by environmental contingencies and events.

By conceptualizing aberrant modes of responding in children with autism as maladaptive learning strategies that result from an interaction between biological and environmental factors, behavior problems may be demystified. A functional analysis framework provides a technology for understanding the basis for severe behavior problems and a means to develop and evaluate treatment strategies. These points are illustrated in the next section, outlining behavioral approaches that have been used successfully with the population who is autistic.

Communication Training With Children Who Are Autistic

The area of communication training for children with autism has perhaps received the greatest attention in the behavioral literature, which may be attributed to the pivotal and pervasive nature of deficits in this area. For children who do develop speech, peculiarities such as echolalia, pronominal reversal, and bizarre or seemingly meaningless utterances are frequently encountered (Bartak et al., 1975; Kanner, 1943, 1946). Moreover, many children who are autistic never acquire functional speech skills, although they may be able to learn and use alternative and augmentative forms of communication, such as signs, picture symbols, and so on. In recent years, the emphasis in training has shifted from a preoccupation with teaching verbal skills to one of training functional communication skills that may enable the nonspeaking autistic child to assume a more active role in what Garfin and Lord (1985) call "social-communicative interactions."

Because language develops and is used within a social context, the aim of communication training is to improve the quality, frequency, and/or complexity of children's reciprocal interactions. In the past, initial efforts at communication training were directed toward developing or expanding verbal skills. Typically, training sessions were carried out in a clinic or therapy room devoid of distraction, to maximize children's attention. Although many children were able to acquire speech skills in this manner, they had difficulty generalizing what they had learned to other people, instructional material, or settings (Howlin, 1989). Moreover, it was difficult to teach pragmatic or interactive skills (e.g., establishing joint attention, initiating and maintaining conversations) in a contrived setting that excluded family members and peers.

In view of these drawbacks, training is now often carried out under more naturalistic conditions. Some of the strategies that are used to teach communication skills to children with autism involve: (1) allowing children to initiate an exchange or interaction, thus capitalizing on their current focus of attention and interest and reducing their reliance on others to prompt language; (2) teaching skills within an appropriate context to decrease metaphorical or irrelevant language usage; (3) varying environmental factors, such as the setting, people present, and types of material available to enhance generalization of skills and motivation to respond; (4) using naturally occurring reinforcers to promote long-term maintenance of skills; (5) directly targeting social pragmatic skills that form the basis for communicative exchanges, such as waiting and turn-taking; and (6) reinforcing appropriate attempts to communicate, rather than focusing on the "correctness" of the response to maintain motivation and reduce frustration and agitation that may trigger avoidance or escape-related behaviors (Dunlap & Koegel, 1980; Koegel, Koegel, & Surratt, 1992; Koegel, O'Dell, & Koegel, 1987; Rincover & Koegel, 1975).

The following examples illustrate how these various elements may come into play during communication training for children with autism. The first example is a nonverbal autistic child who engages in self-stimulation throughout the day. Initial efforts at communication training may center around child-identified objects or activities that evoke interest. The child is reinforced by being allowed to engage in a preferred activity whenever he or she exhibits an appropriate communicative response, which may involve one or more of the following: (1) a vocalization or verbalization; (2) gesturing, reaching, ·or leading the teacher toward the item; or (3) establishing joint attention by gazing at the teacher and the item. Several highly preferred activities are varied or rotated intermittently to maintain the child's attention and motivation to respond. Pragmatic interactive skills may be trained by incorporating waiting and turn-taking into the routine, with the teacher and the child taking turns engaging in the activities. The child may also be taught more functional uses for toys and items, with the intent of broadening their repertoire of appropriate "play skills" and reducing the amount of time spent engaging in self-stimulation.

A different approach is taken for the high-functioning autistic child who has difficulties initiating and maintaining conversations with family and peers. Deficits in pragmatic skills may be remediated by use of a "script" for social exchanges (Krantz & McClannahan, 1993). The child and the teacher may work together on writing a script for greeting friends and conversing about daily events. The script would provide appropriate comments or questions for the child to initiate and outline strategies for responding to the speaker. The child is enlisted to assume a more prominent role in intervention process, with the aim of teaching the youngster a set of skills and problem-solving strategies that may be generalized to produce widespread improvements in communication and social skills.

Figure 5–7 depicts the effects of using written scripts on the frequency of social interactions by children with autism toward nondisabled peers. Scripts were individualized for each child and consisted of a series of questions or statements that could be used to initiate or maintain a verbal exchange. Children's reliance on the scripts was reduced by gradually fading written prompts until youngsters were able to converse in a more independent and naturalistic manner (Krantz & McClannahan, 1993).

EXTENSIONS

The primary consideration for the application of behavioral psychology research and treatment techniques with persons having developmental disabilities has been to address learning and behavior problems secondary to the primary neurologically based disabilities. One additional application is especially worthy of note here because of the value to children and parents and because it is frequently overlooked. The techniques employed to address behavior and learning problems can also be used to facilitate medical diagnostic and treatment procedures necessitated

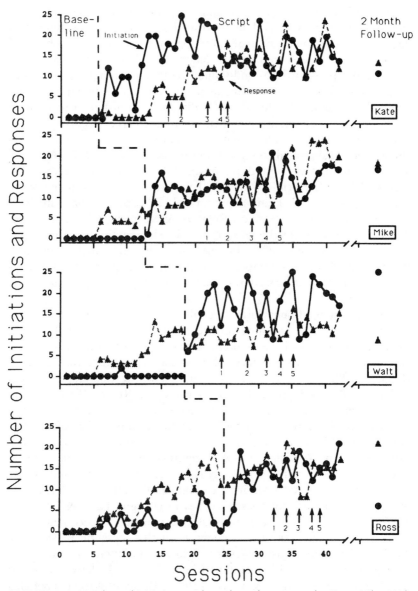

FIGURE 5–7. Number of initiations and number of responses by Kate, Mike, Walt, and Ross during baseline, script, and follow-up sessions in the classroom. Arrows indicate the introduction of fading steps. *From* Krantz, P. J. & McClannahan, L. E. (1993). Teaching children with autism to initiate to peers: Effects of a script-fading procedure. *Journal of Applied Behavior Analysis, 26*(1), 121–132. Reprinted by permission.

by the various sequelae of the primary neurologically based handicaps and syndromes that constitute the broad spectrum of developmental disabilities. The importance of this type of application of behavioral psychology is underscored by the magnitude of these sequelae.

Almost two-thirds of individuals with mental retardation have chronic conditions requiring medical intervention (Minihan & Dean, 1990). For example, up to 50% of individuals with mental retardation have some type of seizure disorder, 30% have cerebral palsy or other motor impairment, 20% have sensory impairments, and 30% have psychiatric or behavioral disorders (McLaren & Bryson, 1987). As many as 33% of individuals with developmental disabilities have feeding disorders (Palmer & Horn, 1978), 22% have urinary or fecal incontinence (Conroy & Derr, 1971), and approximately 22% percent have difficulties with obesity (Fox, Hartney, Rotatori, & Kurpiers, 1985). Yet, quality of medical care for the person with developmental disabilities may be more difficult to provide. In part, this is because of their inability to verbally elaborate symptoms and difficulty cooperating with diagnostic and treatment procedures because of fear or concurrent behavior problems.

Applications of behavioral psychology to increase opportunities for medical care is one last area for the parent and professional to consider. Recent studies have demonstrated procedures to increase adherence and effect outcome of medical intervention in both normal children (Cataldo, 1982; Varni, 1983; Krasnegor, Arasteh, & Cataldo, 1986) and children with developmental delay (Kedesdy & Russo, 1988). Behavioral procedures have been used to assess and treat severe behavior disorders in those who are developmentally disabled, that place children at immediate medical risk, such as self-injury (Iwata, Dorsey, Slifer, Bauman, & Richman, 1982), aggression (Mace, Page, Ivancic, & O'Brien, 1986), and hyperactivity (Pelham, 1982). Behavioral assessment methodology has been used to evaluate the efficacy of drug and/ or behavior therapies for aberrant behavior (Burgio, Page, & Capriotti, 1985), seizure control (Cataldo, Russo, & Freeman, 1979), neuromuscular disorders such as tics, dystonia, torticollis, cerebral palsy (Bird, 1982), and pediatric gastrointestinal disorders (Whitehead, 1986). The management of pain has combined behavioral and pharmacological treatments (Varni, Walco, & Wilcox, 1990). Behavioral treatments also have been developed for pediatric feeding disorders. Treatments include modification for vomiting, food refusal, selective eating, and transfer from gastrostomy to self-feeding (Hyman et al., 1987). Two brief examples illustrate combining behavioral and medical approaches to ensure quality care for persons with developmental disabilities.

Using Behavioral Procedures to Increase Compliance With Medical Regimens

Children undergoing medical or rehabilitation protocols often present behavior problems that interfere with necessary procedures. Such problems are particularly likely in children with developmental disabilities, because they have greater difficulty understanding the procedures and their benefits, may not be able to communicate their fears and discomforts, and often have preexisting behavior disorders. Behavior problems often are strengthened by naturally occurring consequences such as allowing the child to avoid or escape tedious, frightening, and sometimes painful events. This often occurs with children receiving physical therapy after injuries or orthopedic surgery or when adapting to prosthetic appliances such as braces. For example, Varni, Bessman, Russo, and Cataldo (1980) used behavioral procedures with a 3-year-old burn victim. The child developed scar contracture resulting from second- and third-degree burns to her legs and required Jobst stockings, knee extension splints, and range-of-motion exercises. She exhibited chronic pain behavior including crying, screaming, grimacing, rubbing her legs and refusing to stand. Initial assessment indicated that the child used the behavior to obtain staff attention and avoid wearing splints or performing exercises. Treatment consisted of teaching medical staff to provide praise and rewards contingent on participation in therapy while ignoring manipulative pain expressions. As a result maladaptive behavior was eliminated. The child began assisting with splint application, cooperating with physical therapy, and making positive statements about her accomplishments.

Teaching Specific Medical Self-management Skills

If children (including those with disabilities) are exposed to the proper instructional procedures and provided with adequate incentives, they can learn new, sometimes complex skills, allowing them to cope with and to perform their medical regimens. Why not apply these principles to self-care of medical problems? Behavioral psychology specializes in studying and applying learning principles. Recent studies have shown how to train skills as complex as self-insertion of urinary catheters (Parrish, Hannigan, Page, & Iwata, 1989) and self-administered suctioning of a tracheostomy (Derrickson, Neef, & Parrish, 1991), and teaching children to swallow medication in capsule form (Pelco, Kissel,

Parrish, & Miltenberger, 1987). In the last example, teaching pill swallowing, Pelco et al. (1987) taught two 4-year-old girls with chronic illnesses (hyperammonemia and asthma) to swallow capsules required for the oral administration of their medication. This was necessary because of the large quantity of medication required or the unavailability of an effective and palatable liquid form of the medication. Using the behavioral procedures described above, both children were taught first to swallow size-graded candies, then placebo capsules of increasing size until the capsule size required for medication administration was reliably swallowed. In one case this required as little as a single, 75-minute training session. Both children maintained this skill at 6-month follow-up.

This approach has subsequently been successfully employed with children at a variety of developmental and cognitive functioning levels and involves the following steps: (1) observing the child attempting the required behavior and assessing what, if any, of the behavior he or she can perform, (2) breaking the required behavior into teachable components, (3) defining each component for the purposes of measuring performance, (4) using verbal instructions, modeling, contingent praise, tangible rewards, and, if necessary, physical guidance to teach the child to perform the behavioral components, and (5) gradually requiring the child to independently perform an increasing number of components before rewards are given, until the child can perform the entire task with minimal assistance.

CONCLUSION

What we do, how we react to situations, and interact with others, is broadly labeled as behavior. Depending on one's criteria, what another person does may be described as problem behavior or not. From time-to-time, all children have some behaviors that parents and professionals describe as problematic. Statistically, children with developmental disabilities and related disorders are at greater risk for behavior problems than other children.

What constitutes a problem significant enough for intervention, and how that intervention is to be carried out (employing educational techniques, pharmacological intervention, behavior analysis, etc.), should be decided jointly by parents and professionals. The field of behavior analysis offers the option of applying principles of learning to better understand behavior problems and for provision of practical treatment for children and adolescents with developmental disabilities. The body of basic and applied research in the field of behavior analysis for addressing such problems is extensive and offers a sound basis for both individual case and large group applications.

The basic technology for addressing behavior problems employed by behavior analysis views behavior as objective environmental events that are influenced by consequences of the events. This analysis considers the observable definitions of behavior that are the targets for therapy and the antecedent and consequent stimuli that temporally surround these behaviors.

A primary method by which this technology is employed is to objectively define behavior and then quantify it over time and across treatment conditions. The graphic display of such data is typically done in a way that can be readily understood by those outside the field of behavior analysis, including other professionals and parents, so that all may judge treatment effects and share in treatment decisions. Typical graphic methods employed to judge treatment effects include reversal and multiple baseline aproaches. These are used to increase confidence that desired behavior changes are caused by the treatments.

Successful applications of research in behavior analysis and the resulting technology range across a wide variety of problems, including toilet training and other self-help skills, the development of a range of adaptive behaviors, and the reduction of severe and dangerous behavior such as self-injury and aggression. Both overt molar-type behaviors, as well as physiological responses, can be defined and modified by behavioral techniques. Therefore, problems such as neuromuscular control, fecal incontinence, and a variety of other physiological responses have been the subject of research and treatment studies, including persons having developmental disabilities.

Lastly, behavior analysis can be an effective tool in helping other disciplines carry out basic assessment and treatment approaches. This is particularly an important consideration when the behavioral cooperation of the patient/client is essential to proper assessment and treatment. Techniques and principles from behavior analysis have already been incorporated into the fields of physical and occupational therapy, speech and hearing assessment, speech and language training, special education, and most recently for medical diagnostic and treatment techniques.

Although the field of behavior analysis offers powerful technology for behavior change that can be employed by other professionals, teachers, parents, and so on, it is an area that is most successful when integrated with techniques from other disciplines. This is an especially important consideration for problems related to developmental disabilities, because causes and sequelae are complex and can only best be addressed by understanding deficits from a variety of different professional viewpoints.

CHAPTER 6

CHILDREN WITH DEVELOPMENTAL DISABILITIES: FAMILY ISSUES

Nick Elksnin, Ph.D., NCSP
Linda K. Elksnin, Ph.D.

$\mathbf{A}$s discussed in the previous chapters, behavioral/emotional issues and issues that take place within the family are secondary to, that is derivative of, primary neurologically based disabling conditions. It will be necessary to understand family issues in order that we are able to place working with the child with developmental disabilities into the proper context. In our discussion of families of children with disabilities we take a family systems perspective. This perspective is consistent with Public Law 99-457 (1986), the Infant, Toddler, Preschool Act of 1986 (P.L. 99-457). In one of 14 requirements for providing appropriate services, the act requires the development of an individualized family service plan (IFSP). The IFSP is developed through assessment of: the child's strengths and weaknesses in the areas of physical, cognitive, language and speech, psychosocial, self-help skill development; *and* the family's strengths and needs as relating to enhancing the child's development. The IFSP acknowledges the unique relationship of the family to the young child, which must be considered if we are to develop appropriate services. This position is reflected in Public Law 101-476, the Individuals with Disabilities Act (IDEA) of 1990, which requires parental involvement in the development of the child's individualized education plan (IEP).

The primary tenet of family systems theory is that an individual can best be understood within the context of the family. This thinking is a direct departure from that of psychologists and counselors in the 1950s, who focused attention on the diagnosis and treatment of the individual in isolation. In the sections that follow, we draw heavily on the work of Lambie and Daniels-Mohring (1993), who seek to understand children with disabilities within a family systems framework, as well as the contributions of Turnbull and Turnbull (1990). Before we discuss the effects of the child with a disability on the family, we ask the reader to accept these assumptions:

- Families of children with disabilities encounter problems and frustrations that are not faced by families of children without disabilities.
- At the very least, parents and other family members face unique challenges.
- Having a child with a disability, however, does not preclude family happiness and harmony.

Turnbull and Turnbull (1990) suggest that the family of a child with a disability can best be considered as the interrelationship of four variables: family characteristics, family interaction, family life cycle, and family functions.

FAMILY CHARACTERISTICS

Characteristics of the Exceptionality

The type, severity, and demands of a disability will influence family acceptance. Disabilities that are familial; visible; affect the central nervous system, eyes, or genitalia; threaten the life of the child; affect the child's future development; require repeated hospital or agency visits; and present multiple signs may be perceived more negatively than other disabilities by parents (Irvin, Kennel, & Klaus, 1982).

Characteristics of the Family

It is important to consider that individual family characteristics may have concomitant negative and positive effects. For example, lower socioeconomic status families generally view the birth of a child with a disability as requiring the reorganization of the family and extension of roles rather than as a tragic event. Because higher socioeconomic status families tend to place more emphasis on achievement potential, they may regard the birth of a child with a disability as extremely tragic. However, more affluent families report feeling more in control of the situation and the environment than their less affluent counterparts. Family characteristics reported to affect reactions either positively or negatively include number of children in the family, previous births of children without disabilities, the birth order of the child with the disability, and if the family has one or two parents. The ages, levels of education, religiosity, and cultural attitudes of the parents also affect reactions. Personal characteristics such as health of family members and their coping styles play a part as well. Finally, the cultural background of the family may exert an influence on reactions to having a child with a disability.

Cultural Differences

The population of the United States has changed radically over the last several decades (Harrison, Sarafica, & McAdoo, 1984 in Seligman & Darling, 1989):

Group	Percent of the Population
Afro-Americans	11.6
Hispanics	6.4
Asian, Pacific	1.4
Native Americans	.6
Whites	80.0

For professionals to provide appropriate services to children with disabilities and their families, we must acknowledge and accept ethnic differences, acknowledge our own culture, recognize the dynamics of cultural differences, possess knowledge about a family's culture, and adapt our skills accordingly (Cross, 1988). We need to avoid stereotyping ethnic and cultural groups, yet recognize that cultural differences exist. The effects of these cultural differences become apparent in the following examples.

Although many characteristics attributed to Afro-American subculture are economically rather than culturally based, several attributes of this subcultural emerge, irrespective of socioeconomic status (SES) (Seligman & Darling, 1989). These characteristics include spirituality, communalism, harmony, orality, movement, affect, expressive individualism, verve, and social time perspective. In addition, the subculture recognizes the influence of the institutional religion and the importance of the extended family and the community. These extensive support networks may be important resources for the Afro-American family of the child with a disability. Conversely, some evidence suggests that the value placed on early independence, may cause these families to be negatively affected by a child with developmental delays.

Characteristics of the Mexican-American subculture that differ from those of the Anglo-American culture include an emphasis on being rather than doing, present rather than future time orientation, cooperation rather than competition, less emphasis on materialism, and a fatalistic attitude (Seligman & Darling, 1989). These values may enable Mexican-American parents to be more accepting of the child with a disability than Anglo parents. These parents generally are more concerned with individuality rather than the child meeting developmental milestones, although this attitude may lead parents to be overprotective. The professional must recognize the influence of the extended family. For example, a physician's diagnosis and treatment recommendations are likely to be discussed and accepted or rejected by all family members. For a detailed discussion of how ethnic and cultural difference affect working with children with disabilities and their families, the reader is referred to Nazzaro (1981).

FAMILY INTERACTION

Interaction among family subsystems affects the family's ability to accept the child with a disability. Family systems theory recognizes four subsystems. These include the *spousal subsystem* (i.e., husband-wife interactions), the *parental subsystem* (i.e., parent-child interactions), the *sibling subsystem* (i.e., child-child interactions), and the *extrafamilial subsystem* that includes interactions by the whole family or individual family members with friends, neighbors, extended family members, and professionals (Minuchin, 1974). Family systems theory recognizes the importance of system boundaries and systems are regarded as functioning well when there is *cohesion* of subsystems and boundaries are clear and semipermeable. Dysfunctional boundaries are those that are either too rigid or too blurred. When subsystems become *enmeshed,* their boundaries become blurred and overinvolvement and overprotection can result. Subsystems are described as *disengaged* when boundaries are rigid and little communication occurs between members. It is important to acknowledge that most families fall in the middle of the continuum and that a family's position on the continuum is dependent on the age of the child. For example, nurturing the adolescent requires more disengagement, as family members allow the child to gain greater autonomy and independence.

Besides subsystem cohesion, we also are concerned with a family's *adaptability*, or ability to respond to changing circumstances with some degree of flexibility. Viewed as a continuum, families may fall at one extreme and be characterized as *rigid*. Roles within rigid subsystems are narrowly defined and the family operates according to strictly enforced rules administered within a hierarchical power structure. At the other extreme are families characterized as *chaotic*, in which roles are ambiguous and rules are nonexistent or rarely enforced. In the sections that follow we briefly discuss effects a child with a disability may have upon each of the four family subsystems.

The Spousal Subsystem

There is substantial evidence that suggests having a child with a disability places stress on a marriage (Gargiulo, 1985). Couples may have little time or energy to nurture their relationship as they juggle their time and energy to meet the needs of the child, the needs of other siblings, and job demands. It is also important to remember that the functions of the spousal subsystem may be assumed by a single parent or a parent and a significant other.

The Parental Subsystem

The parental subsystem fulfills the functions of nurturing and disciplining. Roles may be assumed by biological or adoptive parents, parent and grandparent, parent and stepparent, or single parent. Nurturing of the child with a disability can only occur after acceptance, which will be discussed later in this chapter. Fostering independence may be difficult when developmental progress is unclear. For families to function adequately, parents must reach consensus about discipline. If the mother assumes primary responsibility for the child with a disability, she may view the child's behavior differently than the father. Parents of the child with special needs also may be confused about what the child can do.

Professionals can help these parents by providing information about support groups and parenting classes.

The Sibling Subsystem

The sibling subsystem carries out the tasks of socialization and development of the children in the family. In families that do not have children with disabilities, parental attention usually is distributed across siblings. The child with special needs may receive a disproportionate share of parental attention leading to resentment, jealousy, and hostility from brothers and sisters. A nondisabled sibling may be expected to assume parenting functions. Some nondisabled siblings may experience "survivor's guilt" and experience stress, as this feeling is rarely shared with parents. Finally, siblings may experience many reactions reported by parents of children with disabilities, including guilt, grief, fear, shame, embarrassment, and rejection. However, when parents' adjustment to the child with special needs is healthy, nondisabled siblings may experience some positive effects, including enhanced tolerance toward individual differences.

The Extrafamilial Subsystem

The extrafamilial subsystem enables the family to interact with the outside world. This subsystem provides emotional support and resources, as well as support for the family's value system. It also is a source of social and recreational activities. Other family subsystems may be affected in a variety of ways by the extrafamilial subsystem. The spousal system may be negatively affected if only one spouse is involved in support groups, or if a spouse is overinvolved with his or her family of origin. The relationship may be strengthened and nurtured if both spouses enjoy the support of extended family. As professionals, our interactions with the parental subsystem may be positive or negative. At its best, the interaction permits professionals to provide support to parents and to model appropriate parenting behavior. Extrafamilial-sibling subsystem interaction is essential if the special needs child and his or her siblings are to acquire social skills and a positive self-concept.

Families of children with disabilities may have smaller extrafamiliar networks as they sometimes withdraw from support networks. Sometimes friends and families withdraw from a family including a child with disabilities because they are unsure how to provide help and support.

FAMILY FUNCTIONS

Turnbull and Turnbull (1990) have identified seven family functions: economic, daily care needs, recreation needs, socialization needs, self-identify needs, affection needs, and educational-vocational needs. As professionals we can assist families of children with disabilities in fulfilling each of these functions.

Economic Functions

All families must generate income and make decisions about how it will be spent. Families of children with disabilities often have greater economic demands placed upon them and may suffer from reduced earning capacity because of caregiver demands. For children with severe disabilities families must contend with medical costs. Families of children with milder disabilities may also face funding services such as tutors, educational materials, medication, and so forth. An additional stressor is planning for the future of the child with a severe disability. Professionals can help families by providing information about financial assistance (i.e., Social Security disability benefits, Medicaid, etc.), suggesting resource persons who can help with financial planning or helping them contact support groups.

Daily Care Needs

The day-to-day demands of cleaning, doing the laundry, cooking, and so forth may become even more acute for the family of a child with a disability. Depending on the age of the child and the nature of the disability, parents may assume caretaking responsibility much longer than other parents. There is some evidence to suggest a direct relationship between the amount of caregiving and the stress level of parents. Professionals can help parents by putting them in touch with agencies and organizations that offer respite care. Educators can work closely with parents to teach the child with disabilities appropriate self-care skills such as dressing, toileting, and feeding, as well as skills that can help the family, such as folding laundry, setting the table, and taking out the trash. Finally, as professionals we need to remind parents of children with disabilities that they have their own mental and physical health needs.

Recreation Needs

The social and recreational activities of some families of children with disabilities may be fewer than those of other families. Turnbull and Turnbull (1990) point out that the family's ability to have recreational breaks makes a major contribution to its mental health. Professionals can provide information about community-sponsored activities and encourage parents to foster the recreational interests of the child with a disability.

Socialization Needs

A common characteristic of children with disabilities is poorly developed social skills that interfere with their relationships with peers and adults and may adversely affect their vocational development. Families need to provide opportunities for these children to practice using social skills. Parents themselves may have difficulty maintaining friendships and developing new ones if they are embarrassed by their child with a disability; or caregiving responsibilities may make it difficult for parents to have the opportunity to socialize at all. However, support groups may enable parents to form long-lasting friendships. Professionals can help parents become more confident by suggesting resources such as parenting classes or by modeling procedures parents can use to more effectively manage their child. Informing parents about appropriate support groups may also be helpful.

Self-identity Needs

The family influences the individual's perception of and feelings about self. Parents may experience loss of self-worth and self-confidence with the birth of a child with a disability or if an older child with special needs fails to respond to discipline. The identity of siblings may be sharply influenced by families engrossed in the disability with few outlets other than participation in support groups, home intervention programs, advocacy activities and so forth. Brothers and sisters may have difficulty separating themselves from the disability and may even fear they can "catch it." Professionals can help by encouraging family members to pursue their own activities and interests and by pointing out that the special needs child needs opportunities to make choices and to assume leader as well as helper roles.

Affection Needs

Families need to provide unconditional love to the child with special needs. The ways in which they show love and affection influence relationships siblings develop outside the family. Some families may have difficulty expressing affection toward the child with a disability because of physical characteristics. Family members may resist forming a strong emotional bond because they fear the child's death. A particularly sensitive topic is the emerging sexuality of the child with a disability. Professionals can support families in meeting their affection needs by recognizing these needs are as important as physical and educational needs. Professionals can offer information and link families with appropriate resources and support groups.

Educational and Vocational Needs

Professionals need to recognize that educational and vocational needs are among the many needs of the family. As professionals we also must recognize that the value families' place on education may differ from our own. Turnbull and Turnbull (1990) caution well-meaning professionals from taking a "fix it" approach to working with children with disabilities and their families. Such an approach results in every situation being turned into a teaching opportunity. We need, however, to emphasize the importance of appropriate education and providing parents with information about programs and support resources. The literature suggests that family decision making is strongly influenced by the expectations of professionals. We need to raise family expectations as well as encourage families to allow the child with the disability to gradually assume greater decision-making responsibilities.

FAMILY LIFE CYCLE

Lambie and Daniels-Mohring (1993) describe six stages of the normal family life cycle. They suggest that each of the stages features a *plateau period* of relative stability and a *transitional period* that occurs when the family must change its structure or function in response to a life event. Events that are most stressful are those that do not occur at expected points in the life cycle, such as the death of a spouse at an early age or the birth of a child in middle age. Each stage has primary themes that require the family to engage in appropriate developmental tasks (Kantor, 1983). Having a child with a disability can affect each stage of the life cycle.

Stage 1: The Newly Married Couple

The primary theme during this stage is attachment. Tasks include committing to the marriage through the development of common goals and realigning relationships with family and friends to include the new spouse. If either member of the new couple is the sibling of a child with a disability, there may be concerns regarding how extended family members will react. A sibling with a disability may affect the couple's planning for the future, including their decision to have children of their own, if the disability is genetically transmitted.

Stage 2: Families with Young Children (Ages 0-5)

During this stage, the theme is industry and the development of strategies to accomplish goals. Tasks include adjusting the marital and extrafamilial systems to include children, developing parenting styles, and adjusting sexual relationships. Parents of children with disabilities diagnosed at birth go through stages of adjustment that will be discussed later in this chapter. In addition, mother-infant bonding and attachment may be hampered, if the child is hospitalized in the neonatal intensive care unit for extended periods. Child care demands of infants who are unresponsive significantly elevate parents' stress levels. As professionals we need to provide families with information, resources, and emotional support to help parents deal with these issues.

Stage 3: Child Rearing Families (Ages 6-12)

Kantor (1983) identifies affiliation and inclusion, consolidation of achievements, and integration of others within the family as the primary themes during this stage. Tasks include establishing sibling roles, involving child peers, and dividing family responsibilities. Most children with disabilities are diagnosed after they enter school. Professionals can foster a better adjustment by providing parents with information about the disability and helping them in planning appropriate educational services.

Stage 4: Families With Adolescents (Ages 13–19)

The primary theme of families with adolescents is a loosening of boundaries and decentralization. Tasks include facilitating and managing the adolescent's increased independence, increasing role flexibility, and reexamining midlife career and marital issues. As for any family, this is the most difficult stage for families of children with disabilities. Adolescents face major physical and emotional adjustments, complicated by the disability. Families need assistance in planning for the future.

Stage 5: Families Launching Children (Ages 20 and over)

Themes of this stage are detachment and differentiation. Developmental tasks include renegotiating roles with adult children, reexamining the spousal relationship, and realigning the system to include in-laws of married children. Children with disabilities should be encouraged by parents to become as independent as possible. Parents and an adult child with disabilities confront employment and community integration issues.

Stage 6: Families in Later Life

Themes include dissolving ties and letting go. The family must redefine roles and confront the deaths of family and friends. Parents have the added task of ensuring that the child a disability will be cared for and supported after their deaths.

STAGES OF PARENTAL REACTION TO DIAGNOSIS OF DISABILITY

Much has been written about parental reactions to the diagnosis of a disability. Parents experience a cycle of grief when the birth of a child with a disability shatters the myth of the perfect child. Reactions are mediated by individual reasons for having a child in the first place, which may include extending self, fulfilling dreams through the child, presenting a gift to a spouse or grandparents, or demonstrating parenting ability. The birth of a child with a disability results in a discrepancy between parental expectations and reality that may be difficult to resolve.

For many years, professionals viewed parents as progressing in lockstep through reaction stages. We now acknowledge *patterns of parental reactions* and view stages as fluid, with each parent passing in and out of stages during the adjustment process (Gargiulo, 1985). Besides reactions to the child with a disability, reactions also include those toward family, friends, or oneself, as well as responses to inappropriate treatment by professionals. In the sections that follow, we review parent reactions to early diagnosis of disability using a model developed by Gargiulo (1985). We should acknowledge, however, that each parent's reactions vary and each diagnostic situation is unique. When a later diagnosis is made, parents grieve differently and they may experience relief when their child is finally diagnosed.

The Primary Phase

The initial reaction of parents is one of *shock*, followed by disbelief. *Denial* occurs when parents refuse to accept the disability diagnosis, minimize the disability, or seek out other professionals to counter the diagnosis. A more subtle form of denial emerges when parents become too cooperative with professionals. *Grief, depression, and withdrawal* also are common reactions during this phase. Parents grieve the birth of a child with a disability much as they would the death of a child. Depression or anger turned inward follows. Physical and emotional withdrawal may allow parents to recuperate, but extended withdrawal is counterproductive and may prevent the family from accepting the child with a disability.

Secondary Phase

Ambivalence is a common reaction during this phase. The child with a disability may intensify normal parental emotions of love and anger. Some parents may wish the child were dead and feel guilty about these feelings. A parent may deal with these guilt feelings by assuming a martyr's role that negatively affects siblings and spouse. Emotional pain may be dealt with through rejection that is demonstrated by minimizing the disability, or by developing unrealistically high or low expectations for the child. Parents may meet physical needs but ignore emotional needs by excluding the child from family activities.

Guilt is one of the most difficult reactions for parents to overcome. Parents need to be reassured that guilt is a normal and healthy reaction so they can move beyond it. Parents often speculate that the disability would never have occurred "if only" they had done certain things differently. They may overcompensate, resulting in the disability becoming more important than the child.

Parents experience *anger* following diagnosis. They may rage against the unfairness of the situation and this is a normal, acceptable reaction. Misplaced anger, however, is unproductive. This occurs when parents direct their rage toward physicians, teacher, spouse, or siblings and they must learn to redirect their feelings toward the disability.

Tertiary Phase

One of the last adjustment stages, *bargaining*, occurs when parents attempt to "strike a deal" with God, science, or anyone they feel can cure the disability. As parents become more confident about their parenting skills, they engage in *adaptation and reorganization* as they consider their relationship with the child. Hopefully, parents will reach *acceptance* of and *adjustment* to the child with a disability. As professionals we need to recognize that acceptance and adjustment are ongoing processes and that negative feelings may remain.

OTHER ASPECTS OF PARENTAL REACTION

Gargiulo (1985) describes four additional reactions encountered by parents of a child with a disability.

Chronic Sorrow

Chronic sorrow is almost a universal reaction among parents of children with moderate or severe retardation. It can coexist with acceptance and lasts until the death of the child. Professionals should view chronic sorrow as a legitimate reaction and provide appropriate support and resources as necessary.

Shopping Behavior

Parents have been accused of going from professional to professional or treatment program to treatment program rather than accepting a diagnosed disability. For many years this shopping behavior was regarded by professionals as a pathological response to guilt. Gargiulo (1985) suggests that shopping should be considered as a response to professionals' failure to assist parents in overcoming their sorrow. Professionals fail parents by not suspecting a disability or not informing parents of a disability. More frequently, however, parents fail to hear the professional's diagnosis. Professionals can avoid this by using some guidelines presented at the end of this chapter.

Rejecting Parents

Rejection is expressed by parents in several ways. Parents may underestimate the child's ability or set unrealistically high achievement goals. Some parents escape the situation through desertion or institutionalizing the youngster. Parents may fail to recognize their negative feelings and present themselves as warm and loving, which is called a *reaction formation*. A distinction should be made between *primary rejection* of the disability and the more common *secondary rejection* of the child's behavioral manifestations.

Compensating Parents

Compensation occurs when parents attempt to replace their attitudes of rejection with attitudes of acceptance. Bryant (1971) provides the following example of this substitution:

Acceptance		Rejection		Compensation
Love	+	Indifference	=	Possessiveness
Empathy	+	Selfishness	=	Sympathy
Forgiveness	+	Fault-finding	=	Overpermissiveness
Gentleness	+	Cruelty	=	Smothering
Caution	+	Carelessness	=	Suspicion
Activity	+	Apathy	=	Overactivity

EXPLAINING THE DIAGNOSIS TO PARENTS

Major errors professionals commit when informing parents that their child has a disability include:

- Delay in defining the problem
- False encouragement of parents
- Too much advice on matters such as institutionalization

- Abruptness
- Hurriedness
- Lack of interest
- Hesitancy to communicate (Ehly, Conoley, & Rosenthal, 1985, p. 16)

Turnbull and Turnbull (1990), the parents of a child with moderate retardation, provide the following positive suggestions for explaining a disability to families:

- Provide full and honest information about the condition of the child.
- Repeat the information in many different ways and at many different times.
- Try to tell both parents simultaneously.
- Encourage parents to ask questions.
- Avoid using educational and/or medical jargon as much as possible; explain those terms that must be used.
- Present a balanced perspective—discuss possible positive outcomes as well as limitations.
- Avoid a patronizing or condescending attitude.
- Encourage parents to join a support group or introduce them to a family who is coping successfully with a son or daughter who has a similar exceptionality.
- Realize the parents will need time to consider the diagnosis; set up another conference.
- Allow parents time to express their feelings and be accepting of those feelings.
- Understand that parents may respond with displaced anger; the attack is on the diagnosis, not you.
- If parents respond with anger, avoid being defensive; continue to be supportive and accepting.
- Discuss how to tell brothers and sisters and other family members.
- Suggest reading materials and other resources.
- Assure families that you will be available as a resource to them in the future. (p. 110)

Parents have three primary needs following diagnosis of a disability. Parents need *information* on an ongoing basis. Professionals are more highly valued by parents as information-givers than emotional supporters. Following diagnosis, parents will begin to explore treatment *options*. Parents, particularly in the months following early diagnosis, need to feel that they are in control. Professionals can help them in taking charge of the situation by providing information about diagnosis, prognosis, treatment options, and community resources. Finally, parents have a need for *emotional support*. This may be better provided by extended family and friends. The professional, however, can help families in expanding their support networks, providing information about support groups, or starting groups if they are unavailable. Effective services for the child with developmental disabilities will only occur if parents and professionals continue to forge partnerships (Shea & Bauer, 1991; Simpson, 1990). Working together we can ensure that the child who is disabled reaches full potential. Understanding that family issues are the secondary result of primary neurologically based disabling conditions will asssist us in developing effective services and for facilitating change within families.

CHAPTER 7

THE SPECTRUM OF DEVELOPMENTAL DISABILITIES

Robert G. Voigt, M.D.
Nick Elksnin, Ph.D.
Frank R. Brown, III, Ph.D., M.D.

As discussed in the introductory chapter, the authors of this text share many basic principles in our approach to children with developmental disabilities. Inherent in our definition of developmental disabilities is the understanding that these conditions are derivative of central nervous system damage or dysfunction, and, as such, represent chronic disorders that affect individuals across their lifespan. Primary disabling conditions discussed in earlier chapters include significant degrees of motor (cerebral palsy) and cognitive (mental retardation) dysfunction, as well as less severe disorders such as learning disabilities and attention deficit disorder. Also discussed in earlier chapters is the concept of secondary disabling conditions, including various behavioral and emotional disturbances frequently found in association with and derivative of the primary neurologically based disabling conditions.

For purposes of clarity, in preceding chapters we have discussed primary and secondary disabling conditions as if they occur in isolation. At the same time, we have alluded throughout to the neurodevelopmental principle of associated deficits and have suggested that rarely do dis-abling handicapping conditions occur as pure and isolated entities. We have also expounded the principle that mild degrees of developmental disabilities predominate over more severe forms. Combining these perspectives, we appreciate that the most common presentation of developmental disabilities is that in which a child evidences subtle and diffuse neurological dysfunction, and these subtle, diffuse neurological deficits are accompanied by behavioral and emotional handicapping conditions.

In the case examples that follow, a spectrum of developmental disabilities is presented in which disabilities range from mild (learning disabilities, attention-deficit hyperactivity disorder [ADHD]) to severe (mental retardation, communication disorder, cerebral palsy). In each example, a child exhibits a primary neurologically based chronic disabling condition. In no example, however, does the primary disabling condition exist in isolation. In each example, associated neurologically based, as well as secondary behaviorally and emotionally based dysfunction, are noted. As the case examples illustrate, the more severe the primary underlying handicapping condition, the more likely and the more severe will be the associated neurologically based deficits.

In each case example to follow, the child manifests significant secondary emotional and behavioral disabilities resulting from and in response to, their primary neurologically based chronic disabling conditions. These secondary emotional and behavioral disabilities also range from mild to severe, and their existence and severity depend more on the acceptance of and adjustment to a child's developmental disability rather than to the severity of the primary disability alone. Denial, delay in appropriate diagnosis, and/or inappropriate demands and requirements at school or at home can exacerbate these secondary emotional and behavioral difficulties.

CASE 1

C.W., a 37-month-old female, presented at a regular 3-year follow-up to her primary care physician. The parents expressed concerns about perceived delays in development, especially walking and talking, when compared with her cousins. At the same time, the parents acknowledged frustration in dealing with increasing noncompliance, tantruming, and occasional aggressive behaviors. The mother expressed a desire to return to previous employment, and acknowledged frustration in the need to support the child in the home, as she has been rejected from local day care centers because of lack of toilet training and behavioral problems. As the general care physician listened to these concerns, she had a distinct advantage in having been involved with the family from birth. She knew that the pregnancy and delivery had high-risk factors and how those issues might relate to the parents' voiced developmental concerns. Reviewing her records, the physician noted that C.W. was the 35–36 week gestational product of a mother who had been 31 years old. Two previous pregnancies had resulted in first trimester miscarriages. The labor had been spontaneous and delivery was accomplished within 24 hours of membrane rupture. No fetal distress was appreciated during labor and at delivery there were spontaneous cries and respiration, with Apgar scores of 7 at 1 minute and 9 at 5 minutes.

C.W. had feeding difficulties when her mother attempted breast feeding in the first 2 months. Because of poor weight gain and suck during breast feeding, a switch was made to formula. The poor weight gain persisted after formula substitution. Considering this history of risk factors and the parents' developmental concerns, a neurodevelopmental history and examination were initiated. Generally, this process (which can be followed through Tables 1–2 to 1–4) will, depending on the age of a child, take approximately 1 hour to $1\frac{1}{2}$ hours to complete.

Neurodevelopmental History

The physician initiated C.W.'s neurodevelopmental history by asking the parents to recount a history of details of the developmental course to date, commencing in areas in which the parents were expected to be most observant and reliable as historians. Parents are generally most observant in areas of development that they consider important and that are current and obvious. Within a developmental area, the parents were again asked questions that were deemed most observable and important to them and this was used to select areas of development for which initial neurodevelopmental questions would be asked.

The neurodevelopmental history was initiated when the physician asked the parents to comment on the age at which C.W. first walked and talked (the referring concerns). The parents reported that she had walked at approximately 24 months and indicated she crawled up stairs, yet was unable to pedal her tricycle (pushing it with her feet) at the time of the history. Other history provided included sitting without support at approximately 12 months and pulling to stand at approximately 20 months. When directly asked about overall gross motor development, both parents suggested that they perceived significant delay and clumsiness.

Concerning language development, the parents reported that C.W. had a vocabulary of approximately 10 words, frequently resorted to jargoning, did not put 2-word phrases together and was inconsistent (50% successful) in carrying out 1-step directives without a gesture. She reportedly had her first word emerge at 24 months, and had a specific "mama" and "dada" emerging at approximately the same time. Other history relating to language development suggested that C.W. had been "very quiet" within the first year, had made little in the way of sounds, and did not babble until approximately 12 months of age. The parents volunteered that, "she may have more words than she says," but acknowledged that many utterances were of poor quality. The parents felt that there was a significant delay in language development.

Finally, from a visual perceptual/fine motor standpoint (viewed by the parents as social-adaptive skills such as dressing and feeding) the parents reported that C.W. had begun drinking from a cup around 18 months and had begun using a spoon around 28 months, spilling from both. Although her mother had extended considerable efforts in toilet training, it had been unsuccessful. Additional information volunteered by the parents suggested that C.W. had just recently begun to scribble spontaneously when offered a large-sized crayon.

At the conclusion of the neurodevelopmental history, the primary care physician asked the parents to comment on their appreciation of their child's development across all domains. A summary question, "How old does your child seem in her overall development?" was asked. Although the parents were initially reluctant to quantify their child's delay, they eventually agreed in reporting functioning at an approximate 18-month level or $1\frac{1}{2}$ years below her age.

Neurodevelopmental Examination

Generally, the appreciation of a probable current level of developmental function obtained through a neurodevelopmental history, guides the generalist to the level at which to begin the neurodevelopmental examination (here at a 18-month level). To optimally engage the child, the generalist begins the neurodevelopmental examination with the assessment of visual-perceptual abilities. This is done at a level slightly below anticipated developmental level obtained in the history, so the child can enjoy initial success. It was observed that C.W. could scribble spontaneously (although with an immature grasp on the large-size crayon), but would not imitate a vertical or horizontal line (cf. Figure 1–2). To dissociate inability to perform some of these tasks into fine motor versus visual perceptual domains, the generalist next assesses fine motor interference with visual perception through analysis of ability to grasp and manipulate blocks. C.W. showed curiosity in accepting 3 cubes, but exhibited fine motor clumsiness. Fine motor clumsiness was also evident when she successfully imitated a tower of 3 cubes. She could not imitate a train of 3 cubes (cf. Table 1–4). In her frustration, she knocked blocks from the table.

C.W. could identify only one or two basic body parts. She was approximately 50% successful in executing simple directives unaccompanied by gestures, but was unable to successfully complete any two-part directives. Mature jargon was occasionally evidenced, but no real words were heard. She communicated primarily through gestures and the parents anticipated many of her noncommunicated needs. She evidenced frustration when she was unable to express wants. The parents inadvertently attended indiscriminately to all of her behaviors, both positive and negative.

C.W. was observed to have a wide-based and awkward gait. She ran with poor coordination and, as reported by the parents, lacked the ability to ascend stairs, except by crawling on all fours. These functional aspects of gross motor development were compatible with observations from the physician's traditional neurological examination of variable, predominantly diminished tone in both the upper and lower extremities, trunk and neck.

Discussion: Case 1

Case 1 underscores many neurodevelopmental principles outlined in Chapter 1. C.W.'s parents' chief complaints centered on perceived delays in walking and talking. This reflects that certain aspects of a child's development are more obvious than others-in particular, gross motor function (walking) and expressive language (talking). This case also underscores the importance of how a developmental delay affects the child's behavior and family function. Here, broader family concerns relate to the child's ejection from preschool secondary to behavior and related financial constraints created by the mother's inability to return to the workforce. In essence, for this family, there occurs an important interaction between the primary neurologically based deficits in both motor and cognitive function and in secondary behavioral and family-centered issues.

At the time the parents solicited opinions from their primary care physician regarding their suspicion of delays in their child's development, the physician elected to become what we have termed a developmental "generalist." The physician became a generalist in the sense that she elected to attend to the parents concerns through the advantage of her knowledge of the family and her willingness to carry out initial developmental assessment. The key tools used by the physician generalist were a knowledge of child development, plus the neurodevelopmental history and examination. The physician, through the employment of these tools, could develop a series of hypotheses regarding C.W.'s development that included the areas of motor, cognitive, and social-adaptive skills. More typically, physicians refer out their patients to allied health professionals for initial evaluations. Here, if the physician elects to pursue further detailed evaluation through other disciplines (to possibly confirm her hypotheses), she will have sufficient data to continue to provide a continuity of care for this family.

Comparing the parents' reports of C.W.'s developmental milestones with those listed in Tables 1–2 through 1–4, it is apparent that in all developmental domains (motor, visual perceptual/problem solving, language, social-adaptive behavior), she is exhibiting developmental delays. Specifically, with respect to motor development, C.W. walked at 24 months (versus the anticipated 12 months), sat independently at 12 months (versus 6 months), and pulled to stand at 18 months (versus 9 months). Concerning cognitive development (as evidenced by language and visual perceptual/problem solving skills), C.W. began to make babbling sounds around 12 months (versus anticipated 6 months), had her first word emerging at 24 months (versus 12 months), and had a specific "mama" and "dada" emerging at 24 months (versus 12 months). Concerning social-adaptive behavior, she drank from a cup at 18 months (versus anticipated 9 months), used a spoon at 28 months (versus 14 months), and just recently had begun to scribble spontaneously (18-month level).

The neurodevelopmental history reveals that C.W. has progressed at a rate of approximately 50% of that anticipated for her chronological age, with level of function at examination of approximately 18 months. The consistency of rates reported through the developmental history for the different developmental domains results in increased levels of reliability and validity.

When the generalist combines results of the neurodevelopmental examination with those obtained through the history, reliability and validity of developmental conclusions is further enhanced. Neurodevelopmental examination revealed that, with regard to visual perceptual/problem solving C.W. had scribbled spontaneously (18 months), but could not imitate a vertical or horizontal stroke (below 27 months). She duplicated a 3-cube tower (18 months), but not a 3-block train (below 24 months). Concerning language development, she identified one or two simple body parts (18 months) and was 50% consistent in executing one-step verbal commands (18 months). She was unable to complete any 2-step commands (below 30 months). She jargoned (14 months), but no real words were produced (although the parents reported a vocabulary of perhaps 10 words). In the area of gross motor function, her gait was of poor quality and she could not ascend stairs except on all fours (less than 27 months). She pushed, rather than peddled, her tricycle (less than 36 months). In essence, the neurodevelopmental examination confirmed suggestions from the neurodevelopmental history that C.W. was functioning at an approximate 18-month level in all developmental domains. Consistency between the history and examination (as with consistency across developmental domains) heightens the generalist's confidence in the reliability and validity of conclusions regarding levels of developmental function.

As the generalist analyzes C.W.'s developmental profile, the consistency of developmental delay over time suggests that C.W. manifests the most common pattern of developmental delay described in Chapter 1, specifically that of the "static encephalopathy." Knowledge of this static pattern is important to the physician, as it has implications for treatment, management, and prognosis. In static encephalopathy, there may be limited value in pursuing additional testing (e.g., neuroimaging, electroencephalograms, genetic workups, etc.), as it is anticipated that such information would not establish a precise causation and would not alter the future course of developmental delay or influence the prescriptive program.

Armed with conclusions and perspectives gleaned through the neurodevelopmental history and examination, and reflecting on some of the neurodevelopmental principles outlined in Chapter 1, C.W.'s primary care physician could respond to the parents' chief complaints and provide recommendations for future management. In essence, the parents' most basic questions centered on their perceptions of possible developmental delay, especially in walking and talking. C.W.'s physician confirms the parents' suspicions of delay in these areas and would suggest that delays are more diffuse than indicated in their referring complaints. She would then interpret how these pervasive deficits reflect primary neurologically based conditions and how these will chronically affect the child. When the parents "press" for a diagnosis they will be told that C.W.'s deficits are similar to children with moderate mental retardation and cerebral palsy. The physician will then proceed to answer other, more detailed parental questions, including questions regarding prognosis, therapy, and the like.

In response to the chief complaint of behavior problems at C.W.'s day care and noncompliance with parental requests, her physician might appropriately point up the important relationship between her developmental functioning and limited understanding in these situations. This is not to define her behavior as acceptable or that it could not be made more acceptable within the confines of her developmental limitations. This is to say that appropriate interventions would be needed early on at her developmental level in a way she could understand. The physician generalist would then prescribe appropriate early intervention services to address both the primary neurologically based and the secondary behaviorally and emotionally based conditions.

Given a family systems approach, it is obvious that dealing with secondary issues of behavior facilitates higher levels of positive family interaction. If C.W.'s primary neurologically based condition is approached in a developmentally appropriate fashion, then her resulting appropriate behavior will have a positive effect on other family members. In addition, the parents can be advised of developmentally appropriate approaches to toilet training. Instead of the mother feeling like a "failure" trying to toilet train C.W., she can feel successful.

CASE 2

Our first case illustrates the role of the physician generalist in facilitating the early recognition of preschool-age children with significant developmental disabilities such as mental retardation and cerebral palsy. This second case illustrates how a physician generalist can also help in the interdisciplinary identification and management of older children with more "mild" developmental disabilities, such as learning disabilities and ADHD. Neurodevelopmental dysfunction in these situations is more subtle and typically not noted until school age. As a result, children with learning and attentional problems are often first identified by school personnel and subsequently referred to the primary care physician. The physician will again use a neurodevelopmental history and examination to contribute to the diagnostic and prescriptive process, and can help the family as a generalist to ensure a balance of professional perspectives when establishing a remediation program.

Evaluation of Presenting Concerns

W.C. was a 9-year-old male who presented to his primary care physician at the suggestion of his school with concerns regarding learning difficulties and possible ADHD. He was 4 months into third grade programming and his parents voiced concerns about failing grades, excessive motor activity, poor impulse control, inattentiveness, oppositionalism, and aggressiveness. They indicated that W.C. had deteriorating self-esteem, was becoming increasingly socially withdrawn, had poor peer interactions, and was developing significant negativity toward school.

As the physician reflected on these parental and school concerns, he was aware that a prime motivation for parents and school personnel to seek his assistance was their desire for pharmacologic intervention with behaviors. The physician, having incorporated the basic neurodevelopmental principles outlined in our introductory chapter, appreciated that deficits of attention span and impulse control (ADHD) are part of a broader spectrum of primary neurologically based disorders, including specific learning disabilities, fine and gross motor dyscoordination, and deficits of speech articulation, among others. As such, the physician resisted a course of early and premature medication and proceeded to evaluate W.C.'s broader neurodevelopmental and behavioral profile through a neurodevelopmental history and examination.

As in Case l, the physician generalist will use the neurodevelopmental history and neurodevelopmental exam to tease out the primary neurologically based disabling conditions and to ascertain which behaviors are likely to be derivative of these conditions. In the school-age child at-risk for learning disabilities and/or ADHD, the physician attempts to identify neurodevelopmental findings, which, although not pathognomonic for learning disabilities or ADHD, nevertheless correlate quite highly with and are risk factors for subsequent development of these mild developmental disabilities. As always, the neurodevelopmental history begins with an analysis of risk factors occurring during pregnancy, labor, and/or delivery and will help identify any patterns of slowness in subsequent development. With school-age children, the neurodevelopmental history needs to be expanded to include a school history, which includes present and past educational curricula and attempts at remediation. The neurodevelopmental history should also include a history of behavior problems both at home and school, and a family and social history needs to be obtained to identify any family history of learning difficulties or any psychosocial stressors at home that may be at the root of the school problems for the child. Finally, the neurodevelopmental history may well review materials provided by the school to compare the school's view of the child's difficulties with the parents' views.

Neurodevelopmental History

W.C. was the full-term son of a 28-year-old, gravida 3 para 2-3 mother. This pregnancy was complicated only by a case of the "flu" at the end of the first trimester, for which the mother had not been hospitalized. Labor and delivery were uneventful. The mother, in retrospect, did report that W.C. was "more active" in utero than his two older siblings.

No resuscitative measures were required after birth, and mother and baby were discharged from the hospital at 2 days post partum.

W.C. was described by his mother as a "very difficult baby." He was remembered as "colicky," difficult to console, and the mother reported difficult sleep patterns. She said that, as an infant, W.C. never napped and he frequently woke up during the night until almost 3 years of age.

W.C. had difficulties with "spitting up" as an infant, necessitating multiple formula changes. His medical history was notable only for several broken bones and multiple lacerations requiring stitches that had resulted from impulsive behavior, such as climbing high fences and falling off.

W.C.'s family history was notable for a history of school difficulties in his father. W.C.'s father reported that he always had trouble concentrating and following directions at school and always had difficulties with reading. He continued to be a poor reader and he did not read for pleasure. Both W.C.'s older sisters were honor students. W.C.'s parents admitted that they have high expectations for W.C.'s school performance as well and acknowledged disappointment and frustration with his school difficulties. W.C.'s father did, however, identify with his son's problems and he felt that the mother had been strict with W.C., feeling that she had placed inappropriate demands on the child. The parents often argue about what to do about W.C.'s school difficulties and behavior problems, and marital discord has reached a significant level, with the parents having just begun some marital counseling.

The physician generalist next proceeds with the neuro-developmental history, focusing on any quantitative or qualitative delays in preschool development. As in Case 1, the physician initiates the neuro-developmental history by attempting to build the parents' confidence as historians by asking them to recount their child's development in developmental domains in which they are expected to be the best observers. (In the older, school-aged child, the parents often have difficulty in recapping developmental milestones, because milestones occurred in the distant past and deviance in neurodevelopmental functioning is often quite subtle.) The physician begins the neurodevelopmental history by having the parents relate information about events perceived as major events in their child's life, which are usually gross motor, expressive language, and social adaptive skills.

W.C. walked independently at 9 months of age. The parents report that he ran soon after, probably just after 1 year of age. With increased mobility he had become more difficult to handle at home, as he was constantly getting "into everything." Once he was able to walk, the parents report that he had subsequently "never sat still." He pedaled a tricycle at 2 years of age and rode a two-wheeled bicycle without training wheels at $4\frac{1}{2}$ years of age. Despite this history of precocious gross motor development, the parents expressed concerns about awkwardness and clumsiness. Both parents felt that W.C.'s gross motor skills were below average for his age. The father expressed particular dismay with his son's performance at sports, as he had little success in his Little League baseball and soccer games.

This history of gross motor development illustrates the importance of obtaining a qualitative as well as quantitative neurodevelopmental history. Although W.C.'s gross motor milestones are quantitatively within normal limits, he, nevertheless, exhibits significant difficulties with his gross motor performance. This documentation of qualitative rather than quantitative gross motor difficulties illustrates the inherent difficulty in detecting subtle but still significant levels of motor, as opposed to cognitive, dysfunction. Because it is difficult to detect relatively small, but clinically significant levels of motor dysfunction, we probably underestimate the true incidence of motor disability.

From a language standpoint, the parents report that W.C. was using a specific "mama" and "dada" before 1 year of age. They felt that he was putting two words together by 18 months of age, and relating experiences using complex syntax by age 3. The parents describe W.C. as a "chatterbox," talking excessively since he was first able to speak. Despite this history, W.C. did experience some articulation problems, with speech intelligibility affected by rapid rate of production. The parents reported that they did not understand 100% of what W.C. had been saying until he was $4\frac{1}{2}$ years of age. W.C. required speech and language therapy in both kindergarten and first grade. Also, despite his apparent loquaciousness, the parents reported that W.C. often has trouble finding the correct word to use to express what he wants to say. The parents also expressed concerns that W.C. has never seemed to "listen," nor is he able to follow directions any more complicated than 1-step, ungestured commands. They also felt they have to repeat instructions several times, even when they are certain W.C. is paying attention to what they say.

Again, this history of language development illustrates the importance of eliciting a quantitative as well as qualitative neurodevelopmental history. W.C.'s language development appears quantitatively generally within normal limits. He does evidence, however, delays in speech articulation and possibly some subtle difficulties with language processing.

From a visual perceptual/fine motor standpoint, W.C. had no history of problems drinking from a cup or spoon feeding. He still, however, had difficulties cutting with a knife, could not tie his shoes, and exhibited "illegible" handwriting. He was potty trained at $2\frac{1}{2}$ years of age, but continued to wet the bed several times a week. He was unable to negotiate snaps until about 2 years of age, could not unbutton until 4 years of age, and did not master buttoning until 5 years of age.

With the school-aged child, the neurodevelopmental history needs to be expanded to include some information regarding school history. W.C. began school at age 5 in kindergarten. His parents recall that at the end of the first month of kindergarten, they were notified at a parent-teacher conference that he was having difficulties sitting still, getting up out of his seat, talking out of turn, not following directions, and touching other kids. Although he appeared to grasp the academic material presented in kindergarten, he repeated kindergarten secondary to "immature behavior." His problems with inattention and classroom disruption persisted throughout his second year of kindergarten, first grade, second grade, and so far in third grade. He has passed first and second grade academically, although his grades have always been "borderline" across the board. He was described as not having any really close friends, and his parents feel that other kids are wary of him as he "intrudes on their space."

In third grade, W.C. had shown increasing difficulties with academics. His grades were failing in all subject areas. Coinciding with this academic difficulty, his behavior problems had intensified. He appeared more oppositional and was engaged in increasing "class clown" behaviors as attention-seeking devices to avoid doing his school work. In addition, he had withdrawn from his peers and had become more aggressive toward them. He was having increasing difficulties with turning in incomplete assignments and losing his homework. He had been required to stay in at recess and to stay after school to complete work that was not completed during class periods. He had appeared more frustrated with his inability to complete the work and had become increasingly negative about school, especially as privileges were being denied. Although he had once looked forward to going to school, he had attempted to miss school several times in the third grade by feigning illness.

The parents reported that it took "forever" for W.C. to complete his homework. His mother served as tutor at home. She felt that he was easily distracted from his assignments, but also that he often did not quite understand what was expected of him. He had grown to dread his homework time as his primary interaction with his mother had been in the role of tutor. This had caused a marked negative change in the relationship between mother and son.

Information provided by the school reinforced the parents' history of W.C. having problems with inattention, poor impulse control, and excessive motor activity. It also reflected the oppositional and attention-seeking behaviors as described by the parents. In addition, W.C.'s teacher reported that she felt that W.C. was "unmotivated" to learn. She stated in her report that if W.C. would "just sit still and pay attention," that he would do much better at school. As of yet, the school had not performed any psychoeducational testing and W.C. receives no special help at school. The parents reported that the school hoped that W.C. would be placed on medication to improve school performance, so that he would not have to undergo comprehensive psychoeducational testing.

Neurodevelopmental Examination

As with the neurodevelopmental history, the physician generalist uses the neurodevelopmental exam to look for neurodevelopmental findings that correlate with learning difficulties. The neurodevelopmental exam assesses visual perceptual development using drawing and block assembly, assessment of short-term memory using digit and sentence repeats, and uses a traditional neurologic exam that also monitors for soft neurologic signs. The physician performing a neurologic examination with a child's developing nervous system is faced with neurologic findings that are on a developmental continuum-that is, they appear and disappear with development and maturation of the nervous system. Pathology here does not equate simply with the presence or absence of physical findings, but will depend on the extent of their presence and the timing of appearance and disappearance. These soft neurologic signs can have high interexaminer reliability and presence may correlate significantly with learning disabilities.

Throughout the neurodevelopmental exam, W.C. was very talkative and he exhibited excessive motor activity. His work style could best be described as impulsive.

From a visual perceptual standpoint, W.C. could replicate Gesell drawings adequately at a 7- to 8-year-old level. However, he markedly distorted the Union Jack figure (Figure 1–1) at a 6-year-old level, approaching this in a fragmented fashion of a series of small triangles. This performance underscores that it is imperative that the physician observe the child while replicating the figures, as satisfactory replication is not the only information to be obtained. It is important to analyze the child's approach to replication of figures, including such issues as time to complete the figures, and omission of key elements. Here, W.C. did not appear to understand the gestalt of the Union Jack figure. Unless he had been observed in the drawing process, this qualitative deficit in performance may not have been appreciated. In addition, W.C. was impulsive with his drawings, executing them in a "driven" fashion. These errors of approach and assembly of drawings would have been missed if the drawing process were not observed and only the completed figures inspected. This, again, underscores the importance of delineating the qualitative aspects of the child's neurodevelopmental performance.

W.C. was quite impulsive completing block constructs. When first presented the 10-block staircase (Table 1–5) he hurriedly knocked down the staircase and attempted to replicate it by memory. However, he could not do so until the construct was again presented to him and he was instructed to pay close attention to the detail of the design before again attempting to complete it.

W.C. was noted to have an awkward pencil grip and he dug deeply into the page. Thus, besides visual perceptual concerns, he also was observed to have fine motor difficulties as well.

W.C. could repeat four digits in a forward direction as expected at a $4\frac{1}{2}$-year-old level. He could remember five digits as expected at a 7-year-old level, but he could not relate them in the correct order. Thus, of qualitative importance, it appeared that he had difficulty with sequential auditory memory rather than rote auditory memory. He performed better on reversed digits, reversing three digits as expected at a 7-year-old level. This, again, is of qualitative importance, as children with difficulties focusing attention often perform better when their attention is focused on the more interesting task of reversing digits. W.C. had more difficulty with sentence repeats, having difficulty adequately repeating sentences at even a 4-year-old level. This relative difficulty with sentence repeats as opposed to digit repeats also raises qualitative concerns. Children with language processing deficits often exhibit more problems with memory tasks involving language, such as sentence repeats, as opposed to "nonsense" auditory memory tasks such as digit span.

W.C. was asked to describe his school, his family, his favorite activities, and his pet dog. He did appear to have some difficulty elaborating on his experiences, often giving one-sentence answers. Finally, W.C. also showed some difficulty following simple ungestured commands. The commands often needed to be repeated and he did show confusion of prepositions, as well as confusion with temporal commands.

On traditional neurological examination, W.C. did appear to exhibit mildly decreased tone manifest by lax ligaments and relative pronation of his feet with gait. W.C. could balance on either foot, but he did not exhibit a coordinated hop or skip. He also had difficulties with completing a tandem gait. Further, he exhibited difficulties completing rapid alternating movements and he showed marked mirror and associated movements with sequential opposition of his fingers to his thumb. W.C. also exhibited marked choreiform movements with prolonged motor stance, as well as some arm posturing with stressed gait.

On completion of the neurodevelopmental history and the neurodevelopmental exam, the physician appreciated that W.C.'s problems were not exclusively the result of ADHD. W.C. did have a history of inattention, poor impulse control, and excessive motor activity compatible with ADHD, but these problems did not exist in isolation. He exhibited significant associated deficits, including a history of speech articulation difficulties, qualitative gross motor clumsiness, quantitative and qualitative fine motor and social adaptive difficulties, visual perceptual difficulties, and possible language processing deficits. In addition, W.C. exhibited significant secondary emotional and behavioral difficulties derivative of, and in response to, his primary neurologically based difficulties. These included oppositional and attention seeking behaviors, social withdrawal, decreased self-esteem, school negativity, and stressed family relationships.

W.C.'s difficulties with visual perception and language hinted at possible, as of then undiagnosed, learning disabilities. Learning disabilities frequently become apparent around third grade, as this represents a transition between rote learning and more abstract learning. As W.C.'s behavioral and attentional difficulties had worsened in third grade, these increased difficulties may well have represented secondary behavioral responses to inappropriate demands being placed on him at school. In addition, it is possible that his behavioral difficulties had increased at home secondary to inappropriate demands being placed on him at home by his parents as a result of his being in a "high achieving" family.

With the neurodevelopmental assessment complete, the physician generalist refered W.C. back to his school for comprehensive psychological, educational, occupational therapy, and speech and language assessments. W.C.'s parents were referred to a parenting class to learn how to more effectively deal with W.C.'s negative behaviors. The physician also encouraged W.C.'s parents to engage W.C. in more extracurricular activities. The parents were cautioned to pick those activities that W.C. would be good at to foster his self-esteem. These activities would also serve to improve socialization and peer interactions as well. The physician also advised the parents to have someone else, other than a family member, supervise W.C. with his homework, to preserve W.C.'s relationship with his family.

Results of school generated psychological and educational testing suggested that W.C. exhibited a significant discrepancy between his cognitive abilities and achievement in reading and written language. Resource help was begun and modifications were made in his school programming to work around his learning difficulties. In addition, W.C. began receiving occupational therapy and speech and language services at school. As it was difficult to differentiate how much of W.C.'s difficulties with inattention were secondary to a primary neurologically based attention deficit and how much of these difficulties were secondary emotional and behavioral responses derivative of his primary learning difficulties, it was decided by his physician and parents to forego a trial of stimulant medication, to see how W.C.'s behavior responded to his new school setting and services.

W.C. returned for follow-up with his physician 3 months after the initial visit. The parents reported W.C. was experiencing increased self-esteem, fewer oppositional and aggressive behaviors, better peer interactions, and increased school performance since the educational modifications were made. However, the parents reported that even in a small, resource setting, with demands made appropriate for his neurodevelopmental abilities, W.C. continued to exhibit significant inattentive and impulsive behaviors. Thus, at that time, a trial of stimulant medication was begun.

Discussion: Case 2

This case illustrates several neurodevelopmental principles outlined in Chapter 1, especially the common pattern of diffuse, subtle insults to the central nervous system. This neurodevelopmental principle is expressed in terms of "associated deficits." Children evincing difficulties in one developmental function should be suspected of having difficulties in other developmental functions as well. Until proven otherwise, all children with developmental delays have associated deficits—associated deficits are the rule rather than the exception.

W.C.'s case illustrates how associated neurologically based deficits may be overlooked in children with "mild" developmental disabilities, such as learning disabilities and ADHD. He was referred to his physician, at the advice of his school, for medication to control his attention deficit and behavior. However, to recognize only a patient's learning disability or attention deficit, without appreciating the associated neurologically based deficits that accompany it would clearly be inappropriate. It is postulated that ADHD or learning disabilities existing in isolation would rarely be found. Instead, most children described as having ADHD or learning disabilities possess associated neurologically based deficits, in W.C.'s case consisting of intercurrent gross and fine motor incoordination, articulation difficulties, visual perceptual difficulties, and subtle language deficits.

W.C.'s case also shows how children with developmental disabilities exhibit secondary emotional and behavioral handicaps that can be considered derivative of their primary neurologically based disabling conditions. The presence and severity of these secondary emotional and behavioral difficulties depend on the acceptance of and adjustment to the child's developmental disability, rather than on the severity of the child's underlying neurologically based disabling condition by itself. Early recognition and parental acceptance of the disability, and combined parental and teacher understanding of what demands are appropriate for each child, decrease frustration and anxiety on the child's part. Such a decrease in frustration and anxiety results in decreased emotional and behavioral problems. On the other hand, if a child's disability is not recognized or it is not accepted by a parent or teacher, inappropriate demands will be placed on the child, causing anxiety, frustration, decreased self-esteem, school negativity, social withdrawal, and attention-seeking, aggressive, and oppositional behaviors.

In W.C.'s case, his learning disability was not diagnosed until the third grade, and before this recognition it could be assumed that inappropriate demands may have been placed on him at school. His grade repeat in kindergarten, rather than directly addressing what his learning problems were, only served to hide his difficulties for another year. It does not seem likely that his self-esteem benefited from the grade repeat, and it also does not make sense that his "immaturity" would have been corrected by placing him in a class with younger peers. W.C.'s frustration with his learning difficulties led to increasing oppositional and attention seeking behaviors and significant school negativity in third grade. Inappropriate demands placed on him at home resulted in erosion of his relationship with his mother.

Once W.C.'s learning disability was recognized and appropriate modifications were made in his educational placement, he exhibited marked improvement in his secondary emotional and behavioral difficulties. His self-esteem was bolstered, and his relationships with his family improved. Recognition of the primary underlying handicapping condition, parental and teacher acceptance of his disabilities, and parent and teacher understanding of more appropriate demands were the keys in remediating such secondary emotional and behavioral difficulties. While W.C.'s problems markedly improved with educational modification, even in a small group setting he continued to show difficulties with inattention and poor impulse control. Stimulant medication was added to his treatment regimen at that point. It would have been easier for his physician to prescribe stimulant medication at the beginning because of the parents' and school's history of behaviors consistent with ADHD. However, the physician, with the knowledge that most insults to the central nervous system are mild in extent yet diffuse in distribution, geared his evaluation to look for associated neurologically based deficits, and to tease out the secondary emotional and behavioral problems. If this physician had just prescribed medication, W.C. may well have shown some short-term improvement in his school performance; however, his associated deficits would not have been recognized or addressed. Thanks to his physician's neurodevelopmental assessment, W.C.'s primary disabling conditions, as well as associated deficits, were fully recognized and addressed.

GLOSSARY

abduction   Movement of muscles away from the body or away from the midsection.

adduction   Movement of muscles toward the body or toward the midline.

antecedents   In behavioral analytic terms, events that reliably precede the behavior.

associated deficits   Associated delays in areas other than the primary delay which may be subtle and therefore more difficult to observe.

ataxia   Loss of coordinated muscle movements through diseases of the nervous system.

athetosis   Repetitive, involuntary slow muscle movements.

attention-deficit hyperactivity disorder (ADHD)   Developmentally inappropriate lack of attention with associated poor impulse control and excessive motor activity.

audiogram   A graphical representation of auditory status as it relates to frequency (pitch) and intensity (loudness). This is usually described in Hz (hertz) and dB (decibels).

autistic disorder   A severe form of pervasive developmental disorder with onset in infancy or childhood, characterized by impaired reciprocal social interaction, verbal/nonverbal communication, and restriction of activities and interests.

brain stem evoked response (BSER)   A technique of hearing evaluation frequently utilized with infants and young children who are otherwise unable to cooperate with behavioral measures of hearing acuity. Response to a click stimulus in the ear is recorded from scalp electrodes.

cerebral palsy   A descriptive term meaning significant delays in motor development.

chorea   Involuntary, quick, jerking movements while the muscle is at rest.

communication disorder   A developmental delay manifested in poor connected language understanding and usage.

conductive hearing loss   Impairment caused by malfunctioning of the external or middle ear.

consequences   In behavioral analytic terms, events that reliably follow the behavior.

cruising   Ambulation while holding on to objects such as low table tops; an antecedent to independent walking.

dissociation   The process of systematically looking for the relationship between primary deficits and the resulting component parts, which may be considered secondary. The goal is to determine whether or not inability to complete a task relates to a delay in one area of development versus another. Example: Poor articulation being the result of either low muscle tone (motor) versus low cognitive ability (mental retardation).

dystonia   Severely distorted posture of the trunk, neck, and extremities, reflecting damage to the basal ganglia.

encephalopathy   Any disease process affecting the central nervous system. May be static, progressive, or acute.

family systems theory   A model that assumes the individual can best be understood within the context of the family. This can be likened to a hydraulic theory in that each individual has an effect on the other members of the family unit.

fine motor   Movement using hands and fingers for tasks requiring precision.

fluency disorders   Typically referred to as "stuttering." Characterized by repetitions of speech sound or syllables or blocks to articulation and vocalization.

fronting   One of the phonological processes that can result in the mispronunciation of a word whereby the speech sound is produced more anteriorly in the mouth than is appropriate.

generalist   A diagnostician who utilizes a knowledge of child development, and information from a neurodevelopmental history and neurodevelopmental examination. Although usually a physician, other professionals may assume this role.

gross motor   Movements requiring the whole body for appropriate execution. Transfer of body weight and postural adjustment is involved.

hyperactivity   Excessive motor activity, manifested as excessive running or climbing, difficulty sitting still, or excessive movement in sleep.

hypertonus   Markedly increased muscle tone.

hypotonus   Markedly decreased muscle tone.

IEP   Individualized education plan. A written outline of instructional and therapeutic strategies used for the remediation of a disabled student who is found eligible for special education services by the local education agency.

IFSP   Individualized family service plan. A written outline of instructional and therapeutic strategies developed to meet the infant, toddler, or preschooler needs and those of the family in supporting the child. Usually developed by an interdisciplinary team and the family.

interdisciplinary   Format of shared communications, trust, openness, respect, and interdependence between professionals in establishing a diagnosis or developing prescriptive plans.

learning disability   Condition whereby an individual's academic achievement level (in any specific academic area) is significantly below the level that would be predicted from the level of intellectual ability.

mental retardation   A significant delay in cognitive and adaptive development typically defined as IQ and adaptive behavior quotients two standard deviations below the mean.

minimal brain dysfunction (MBD)   Subtle brain dysfunction in which a child exhibits a mixture of some or all of the following: learning disabilities, language disabilities, other inconsistencies among various cognitive functions, attention deficit disorder, gross, fine, and oral motor dyscoordination.

mixed hearing loss   A mixture of both conductive and sensorineural hearing loss.

neurodevelopmental examination   Examination of the level of development in motor (gross and fine), language (expressive and receptive), visual perception/problem-solving, and social adaptive functioning.

neurodevelopmental history   History of the temporal sequence of development in motor (gross and fine), language (expressive and receptive), visual perception/problem-solving, and social adaptive functioning.

pervasive developmental disorders (PDD)   Disorders characterized by qualitative impairment in the development of reciprocal social interaction, in the development of verbal and nonverbal communication skills, and in imaginative activity.

Public Law 94-142   The Education for All Handicapped Children Act of 1975, which provides for free appropriate education of all children who are disabled, including children who are learning disabled, in the least restrictive educational environment.

Public Law 98-524   The Carl D. Perkins Vocational Education Act of 1984, enables students who are disabled and disadvantaged to access the full range of vocational programs available to individuals who are not disabled.

Public Law 99-457   Education of the Handicapped Amendments of 1986, which provides new incentives for the development of services to young children who are disabled and their families. Stipulates development of an individualized family service plan (IFSP).

pragmatics   The use and understanding of language in social contexts.

primary disabling conditions   Disabling conditions that have a neurological basis, including learning disabilities, speech-language disabilities, gross and fine motor dyscoordination, and attention-deficit hyperactivity disorder (ADHD).

prone   Lying face down.

prosody   The speech sounds of rhythm, stress, intonation, and rate that communicate information regarding the attitudes and intention of the speaker.

reliability   The extent to which a test consistently measures what it measures. This includes consistency over time (test-retest reliability), and consistency across forms of the test (alternate form reliability), or consistency within the test items themselves (internal reliability).

secondary disabling conditions   Disabling conditions that do not have a direct neurological basis, but are the result of primary (neurologically based) conditions that have not been properly managed. The most common are poor self-concept and inappropriate attention-seeking behaviors.

sensorineural hearing loss   Hearing loss directly attributable to neurological damage; generally considered an inner ear problem.

soft neurological signs   Neurological findings that are on a developmental continuum-that is, they appear and disappear with development and maturation of the nervous system. Pathology equates with the extent of their presence and the timing of their appearance and disappearance. Mirror movements and synkinesis represent the most commonly encountered.

supine   Lying face up.

tympanometry   A method of hearing assessment that measures the impedance of the tympanic membrane during the emission of a tone. Tympanometry is sensitive to middle ear pathology, although it is less effective with infants under the age of 6 months.

validity   The extent to which a test actually measures what it purports to measure. A test's validity is determined by how well it samples from the domain of behaviors it was designed to measure (content validity), how well the test correlates with other measures of the same or similar construct (concurrent validity), how well the test predicts future performance (predictive validity), and how helpful the test is in understanding the construct measured (construct validity).

REFERENCES

Abbott, R., & Berninger, V. (1993). Structural equation modeling of relationships among developmental skills and writing skills in beginning and developing writing. *Journal of Educational Psychology, 85,* 478–508.

Abell, M., Bly, L., Hanson, D. Kinney, N., Levine, B., McDermott, S., Salek, B., Staller, J., & Williamson, G. (1978). Movement. In F. Connor, G. Williamson, & J. Siepp (Eds.), *Program guide for infants and toddlers with neuromotor and other developmental disabilities* (pp. 103–128). New York: Teachers College Press.

Allen, D. A. (1988). Autistic spectrum disorders: Clinical presentation in preschool children. *Journal of Child Neurology, 3* (Suppl.), S48–S56.

American Occupational Therapy Association (1987). *Guidelines for occupational therapy services in school systems.* Rockville, MD: Author.

American Occupational Therapy Association (1989). *Guidelines for occupational therapy services in school systems* (2nd ed.). Rockville, MD: Author.

American Psychiatric Association (1980). *Diagnostic and statistical manual of mental disorders* (3rd ed.). Washington, DC: Author.

American Psychiatric Association (1987). *Diagnostic and statistical manual of mental disorders. DSM-III-R* (3rd ed.-rev.). Washington, DC: Author.

Anastopoulos, A. D., & Barkley, R. A. (1988). Biological factors in attention deficit-hyperactivity disorder. *The Behavior Therapist, 11,* 47–53.

Anderson, K. L. (1991). Hearing conservation in the public school revisted. *Seminars in Hearing, 12,* 340–363.

Aram, D. M., & Hall, N. E. (1989). Longitudinal follow-up of children with preschool communication disorders: Treatment implications. *School Psychology Review, 18,* 487–501.

Aram, D. M., & Nation, J. E. (1980). Preschool language disorders and subsequent language and academic difficulties. *Journal of Communication Disorders, 13,* 159–170.

Ayres, A. J. (1989). *Sensory Integration and Praxis Texts.* Los Angeles: Western Psychological.

Azrin, N. H., & Foxx, R. M. (1971). A rapid method of toilet training the institutionalized retarded. *Journal of Applied Behavior Analysis, 4*(2), 89–99.

Bakker, X. (1973). Hemispheric specialization and stages in the learning to read process. *Bulletin of the Orton Society, 23,* 15–27.

Barkley, R. A. (1990). *Attention-deficit hyperactivity disorder: A handbook for diagnosis and treatment.* New York: Guilford.

Baron-Cohen, S. (1988). Social and pragmatic deficits in autism: Cognitive or affective? *Journal of Autism and Developmental Disorders, 18*(3), 379–402.

Baroody, A. J. (1988). Number-comparison learning by children classified as mentally retarded. *American Journal of Mental Retardation, 92,* 461–471.

Bartak, L., & Rutter, M. (1976). Differences between mentally retarded and normally intelligent autistic children. *Journal of Autism and Childhood Schizophrenia, 6*(2), 109–119.

Bartak, L., Rutter, M., & Cox, A. (1975). A comparative study of infantile autism and specific developmental receptive language disorder: I. The children. *British Journal of Psychiatry, 126,* 126–145.

Bateman, B. (1968). *Interpretation of the 1961 Illinois Test of Psycholinguistic Abilities.* Seattle: Special Child Publications.

Bates, E., Bretherton, I., & Snyder, L. (1988). *From first words to grammer: Individual differences and dissociable mechanisms.* New York: Cambridge University Press.

Bates, E., Thal, D., & Janowsky, J. S. (1992). Early language development and its neural correlates. In S. J. Segalowitz & I. Rapin (Eds.), *Handbook of neuropsychology, Vol. 7: Child neuropsychology* (pp. 69–110). New York: Elsevier Science Publishers.

Bayley, N. (1993). *Bayley Scales of Infant Development* (2nd ed.). San Antonio, TX: Psychological Corp., Harcourt, Brace, & Co.

Beery, K. (1989). *The VMI Developmental Test of Visual Motor Integration* (3rd ed.). Cleveland: Modern Curriculum Press.

Benbow, M. (1993, January). Observations for cursive writing skills training. Paper presented at the meeting of Neurokinesthetic Approach to Hand Function and Handwriting, Baltimore, MD.

Benbow, M. (1993, January). Observations of hand skill of the "K & 1" child. Paper presented at the meeting of Neurokinesthetic Approach to Hand Function and Handwriting, Baltimore, MD.

Berninger, V., Mizokawa, D. T., & Bragg, R. (1991). Theory-based diagnosis and remediation of writing disabilities. *Journal of School Psychology, 29*, 57–79.

Bess, F. H. (1993). Early identification of hearing loss: A review of the whys, hows, and whens. *The Hearing Journal, 46*(6), 22–25.

Bird, B. L. (1982). Behavioral intervention in Pediatric Neurology. In D. C. Russo & J. W. Varni (Eds.), *Behavioral pediatrics: Research and practice* (pp. 101–141). New York: Plenum Press.

Bishop, D., & Adams, C. (1990). A prospective study of the relationship between specific language impairment, phonological disorders, and reading retardation. *Journal of Child Psychology and Psychiatry, 21*, 1027–1050.

Blackman, L. S., Bilsky, A. L., Burger, A. L., & Mar, H. (1976). Cognitive processes and academic achievement in EMR adolescents. *American Journal of Mental Deficiency, 81*, 125–134.

Bledsoe, N. P., & Shepherd, J. T. (1982). A study of reliability and validity of a preschool play scale. *American Journal of Occupational Therapy, 36*, 783–794.

Boder, E. (1970). Developmental dyslexia: A new diagnostic approach based on the identification of three subtypes. *The Journal of School Health, 40*, 289–290.

Bogen, J. E. (1969). The other side of the brain. Parts I, II, and III. *Bulletin of the Los Angeles Heurological Society, 34*, 73–105, 135–162, 191–203.

Borkowski, J. G., Peck, V. A., & Damberg, P. R. (1983). Attention, memory, and cognition. In J. L. Matson & J. A. Mulick (Eds.), *Handbook of mental retardation* (pp. 479–498). New York: Pergamon Press.

Brigance, A. H. (1978). *Brigance Diagnostic Inventory of Early Development*. North Billerica, MA: Curriculum Associates.

Brown, A. L. (1974). The role of strategic behavior in retardate behavior. In N. R. Ellis (Ed.), *International review of research in mental retardation* (Vol. 7) (pp. 55–113). New York: Academic Press.

Brown, F. R., III, Aylward, E. H., & Keogh, B. K. (1992). *Diagnosis and management of learning disabilities: An interdisciplinary/lifespan approach*. San Diego: Singular Publishing Group.

Brown, R. (1973). *A first language: The early stages*. Cambridge, MA: Harvard University Press.

Bruininks, R. H. (1978). *Bruininks-Oseretsky Test of Motor Proficiency*. Circle Pines, MN: American Guidance Service.

Bryant, J. (1971). Parent-child relationships: Their effect on rehabilitation. *Journal of Learning Disabilities, 4*, 325–329.

Burgio, L. D., Page, T. J., & Capriotti, R. M. (1985). Clinical Behavioral pharmacology: Methods for evaluation of medications and contingency management. *Journal of Applied Behavior Analysis, 18*, 45–59.

Campione, J. C., Brown, A. L., Ferrara, R. A., Jones, R. S., & Steinberg, E. C. (1985). Breakdowns in flexible use of information: Intelligence related differences in transfer following equivalent learning performance. *Intelligence, 9*, 297–315.

Cantwell, D. P. (1975). A model for the investigation of psychiatric disorders: Its application in genetic studies of the hyperkinetic syndrome. In E. J. Anthony (Ed.), *Explorations in child psychiatry* (pp. 57–59). New York: Plenum.

Carr, E. G., & Durand, V. M. (1985a). Reducing behavior problems through functional communication training. *Journal of Applied Behavior Analysis, 18*(2), 111–126.

Carr, E. G., & Durand, V. M. (1985b). The social-communicative basis of severe behavior problems in children. In S. Reiss & R. R. Bootzin (Eds.), *Theoretical issues in behavior therapy*. San Diego, CA: Academic Press.

Cataldo, M. F. (1982). The scientific basis for a behavioral approach to pediatrics. *Pediatric Clinics of North America, 19*, 415–423.

Cataldo, M. F., Russo, D. C., & Freeman, J. M. (1979). A behavior analysis approach to high-rate myoclonic seizures. *Journal of Autism and Developmental Disorders, 9*(4), 413–427.

Cataldo, M. F., Ward, E. M., Russo, D. C., Riordan, M. M., & Bennett, D. (1986). Compliance and correlated problem behavior in children: Effects of contingent and noncontingent reinforcement. *Analysis and Intervention in Developmental Disabilities, 6*, 265–282.

Catts, H. (1993). The relationship between speech-language impairments and reading disorders. *Journal of Speech and Hearing Research, 36*, 948–958.

Chandler, L. S., Andrews, M. S., & Swanson, M. W. (1980). *Movement Assessment of Infants*. Rolling Bay: WA: Movement Assessment of Infants Publisher.

Chelune, G. J., Ferguson, W., Koon, R., & Dickey, T. O. (1986). Frontal lobe disinhibition in attention deficit disorder. *Child Psychiatry and Human Development, 16,* 221–232.

Coggins, T. E., & Carpenter, R. L. (1979). Introduction to the area of language development. In M. A. Cohen & P. J. Gross (Eds.), *The developmental resource: Behavioral sequences for assessment and program planning* (Vol. 2) (pp. 1–41). New York: Grune & Stratton.

Cohn, R. (1971). Arithmetic and learning disabilities. In H. R. Myklebust (Ed.), *Progress in learning disabilities* (Vol. 2) (pp. 176–194). New York: Grune & Stratton.

Colarusso, R., & Hammill, D. (1972). *Motor-free Visual Perception Test.* Novato, CA: Academic Therapy.

Conley, R. W. (1973). *The economics of mental retardation.* Baltimore: The Johns Hopkins University Press.

Conroy, J. W., & Derr, K. E. (1971). Survey and analysis of the habilitation and rehabilitation status of the mentally retarded and associated handicapping conditions (DHEW publication no. (OHD) 76-21008). Washington, DC: U.S. Government Printing Office.

Cross, T. (1988). Services to minority populations: What does it mean to be a culturally competent professional? *Focal Point, 2*(4), 1–3.

Cummins J. P., & Das, J. P. (1977). Cognitive processing and reading difficulties: A framework for research. *Alberta Journal of Educational Research, 23,* 245–256.

Cummins, J. P., & Das, J. P. (1980). Cognitive processing, academic achievement, and WISC-R performance in EMR children. *Journal of consulting and Clinical Psychology, 48,* 777–779.

Das, J. P., Kirby, J. R., & Jarman, R. F. (1979). *Simultaneous and successive cognitive processes.* New York: Academic Press.

Das, J. P., Leong, C. K., & Williams, N. H. (1978). The relationship between learning disability and simultaneous-successive processing. *Journal of Learning Disabilities, 11,* 618–625.

David, O. J., Clark, J., & Hoffman, S. (1979). Childhood lead poisoning: A re-evaluation. *Archives of Environmental Health, 34,* 106–111.

David, O. J., Clark, J., & Voeller, K. K. S. (1972). Lead and hyperactivity. *Lancet, 2,* 900–903.

Davies, D., Sperber, R. D., & McCauley, C. (1981). Intelligence-related differences in semantic processing speed. *Journal of Experimental Child Psychology, 31,* 387–402.

Day, J. D., & Hall, L. K. (1988). Intelligence-related differences in learning and transfer and enhancement of transfer among mentally retarded persons. *American Journal of Mental Retardation, 93,* 125–137.

DeGangi, G., & Berk, R. (1983). *DeGangi-Berk Test of Sensory Integration.* Los Angeles: Western Psychological Services.

DeGangi, G., & Greenspan, S. (1989). *Test of Sensory Functions in Infants.* Los Angeles: Western Psychological Services.

Derrickson, J. G., Neef, N. A., & Parrish, J. P. (1991). Teaching self-administration of suctioning to children with tracheostomies. *Journal of Applied Behavior Analysis, 24*(3), 563–570.

Detterman, D. K. (1979). Memory in the mentally retarded. In N. R. Ellis (Ed.), *Handbook of mental deficiency, psychological theory and research* (2nd ed.) (pp. 1–62). Hillsdale, NJ: Lawrence Erlbaum Associates.

Diefendorf, A. O., Chaplin, R. G., Kessler, K. S., Miller, S. M., Miyamoto, R. T., Myres, W. A., Pope, M. L., Reitz, P. S., Renshaw, J. J., Steck, J. T., & Wagner, M. L. (1990). Follow-up and intervention: Completing the process. *Seminars in Hearing, 11*, 393–407.

Dunlap, G., & Koegel, R. L. (1980). Motivating autistic children through stimulus variation. *Journal of Applied Behavior Analysis, 13*, 619–627.

Dunn, W. (1981). *A Guide to Testing Clinical Observations in Kindergartners.* Rockville, MD: American Occupational Therapy Association.

Dunn, W., & Campbell, P. (1991). Designing pediatric service provision. In W. Dunn (Ed.), *Pediatric occupational therapy: Facilitating effective service provision* (pp. 139–159). Thorofare, NJ: Slack.

Dunn, L. M., & Dunn, L. M. (1981). *Peabody Picture Vocabulary Test-Revised.* Circle Pines, MN: American Guidance Service.

Ehly, S. W., Conoley, J. C., & Rosenthal, D. (1985). *Working with parents of exceptional children.* St. Louis: Times Mirror/Mosby College Publishing.

Ellis, N. R. (1970). Memory processes in retardates and normals. In N. R. Ellis (Ed.), *International review of research in mental retardation* (Vol. 4) (pp. 1–32). New York: Academic Press.

Ellis, A. W. (1982). Spelling and writing (and reading and speaking). In A. W. Ellis (Ed.), *Normality and pathology in cognitive functions* (pp. 113–146). London: Academic Press.

Ellis, N. R., & Dulaney, C. L. (1991). Further evidence for cognitive inertia of persons with mental retardation. *American Journal of Mental Retardation, 95*, 613–621.

Ellis, N. R., Woodley-Zanthos, P., & Dulaney, C. L. (1989). Memory for spatial location in children, adults, and mentally retarded persons. *American Journal of Mental Retardation, 93*, 521–527.

Ellis, N. R., Woodley-Zanthos, P., Dulaney, C. L., & Palmer, R. L. (1989). Automatic-effortful processing and cognitive inertia in persons with mental retardation. *American Journal of Mental Retardation, 93*, 412–423.

Erhardt, R. P. (1989). *Erhardt Developmental Vision Assessment* (EDVA) (rev. ed.) Tucson: Therapy Skill Builders.

Erhardt, R. P. (1994). *Developmental hand dysfunction: Theory, assessment, treatment* (2nd ed.). Tucson: Therapy Skill Builders.

Erhardt, R. P. (1994). *Erhardt Developmental Prehension Assessment (EDPA)* (rev. ed.) Tucson: Therapy Skill Builders.

Exner, C. E. (1990). In-hand manipulation skills in normal young children: A pilot study. *Occupational Therapy Practice, 1*(4), 63–72.

Exner, C. E. (1992). In-hand manipulation skills. In J. Case-Smith & C. Pehoski (Eds.), *Development of hand skills in the child* (pp. 35–45). Rockville, MD: American Occupational Therapy Association.

Feagan, L. V., Short, E. J., & Meltzer, L. J. (Eds.). (1991). *Subtypes of learning disabilities. Theoretical perspectives and research.* Hillsdale, NJ: Lawrence Erlbaum Associates.

Ferguson, J. M., & Taylor, C. B. (Eds.). (1980). *Comprehensive handbook of behavioral medicine* (Vols. 1–3). New York: Spectrum, 1980.

Feingold, B. (1975). *Why is your child hyperactive?* New York: Random House.

Feldman, D. H., & Adams, M. L. (1989). Intelligence, stability, and continuity: Changing conceptions. In M. H. Bornstein & N. A. Krasnegor (Eds.), *Stability and continuity in mental development* (pp. 299–300). Hillsdale, NJ: Lawrence Erlbaum Associates.

Finney, J. W., Russo, D. C., & Cataldo, M. F. (1982). Reduction of pica in young children with lead poisoning. *Journal of Pediatric Psychology, 7*(2), 197–207.

Fisk, J. L., & Rourke, B. P. (1979). Identification of subtypes of learning disabled children at three age levels: A neuropsychological multivariate approach. *Journal of Clinical Neuropsychology, 1*, 289–310.

Folio, M., & Fewell, R. (1983). *Peabody Developmental Motor Scales.* Allen, TX: DLM Teaching Resources.

Fox, R. A., Hartney, C. W., Rotatori, A. F., & Kurpiers, E. M. (1985). Incidence of obesity among retarded children. *Education and Training of the Mentally Retarded, 20*, 175–181.

Frith, U. (1989). A new look at language and communication in autism. *British Journal of Disorders of Communication, 24*, 123–150.

Furuno, S., O'Reilly, K., Hosaka, C., Inatsuka, T., Allman, T., & Zeisloft, B. (1990). *Hawaii Early Learning Profile* (4th ed.). Palo Alto, CA: VORT Corp.

Gardner, H. (1983). *Frames of mind: The theory of multiple intelligences.* New York: Basic Books.

Gardner, M. F. (1982). *Test of Visual-perceptual Skills (Non-motor).* Seattle: Special Child Publications.

Gardner, M. F. (1986). *Test of Visual-motor Skills.* San Francisco: Children's Hospital of San Francisco.

Garfin, D. G., & Lord, C. (1985). Communication as a social problem in autism. In E. Schopler & G. B. Mesibov (Eds.), *Communication problems in autism* (pp. 133–151). New York: Plenum Press.

Gargiulo, R. M. (1985). *Working with parents of exceptional children: A guide for professionals.* Boston: Houghton Mifflin Company.

Gazzaniga, M. S. (1975). Recent research on hemispheric lateralization of the human brain: Review of the split-brain. *UCLA Educator, 17,* 9–12.

Gersten, R. M. (1980). In search of the cognitive deficit in autism: Beyond the stimulus overselectivity model. *Journal of Special Education, 14*(1), 47–65.

Gersten, R. M. (1983). Stimulus overselectivity in autistic, trainable mentally retarded, and non-handicapped children: Comparative research controlling chronological (rather than mental) age. *Journal of Abnormal Child Psychology, 11,* 61–76.

Gesell, A., & Amatruda, C. S. (1947). *Developmental diagnosis: Normal and abnormal child development: Clinical methods and pediatric application.* New York: Paul B. Hoeber.

Gillberg, I. C., & Gillberg, C. (1989). Asperger syndrome—some epidemiological considerations: A research note. *Journal of Child Psychology and Psychiatry, 30,* 631–638.

Gittelman, R., Mannuzza, S., Shenker, R., & Bonagura, N. (1985). Hyperactive boys almost grown up. I. Pyschiatric status. *Archives of General Psychiatry, 42,* 937–947.

Goodman, R. (1989). Infantile autism: a syndrome of multiple primary deficits? *Journal of Autism and Developmental Disorders, 19*(3), 409–424.

Gordon, H. W., & Bogen, J. E. (1974). Hemispheric lateralization of singing after intracarotid sodium amylobarbitone. *Journal of Neurology, Neurosurgery, and Psychiatry, 37,* 727–738.

Gordon-Brannan, M., Hodson, B., & Wynne, M. K. (1992). Remediating untillegible utterances of a child with a mild hearing loss. *American Journal of Speech-Language Pathology: A Journal of Clinical Practice, 1*(4), 28–38.

Gravel, J. S., & Stapells, D. R. (1993). Behavioral, electrophysiologic, and otoacoustic measures from a child with auditory processing dysfunction: Case report. *Journal of the American Academy of Audiology, 4,* 412–419.

Green, D. M. (1976). *An introduction to hearing.* New York: Lawrence Erlbaum Associates.

Gregg, N. (1992). Expressive writing. In S. R. Hooper, G. W. Hynd, & R. E. Mattison (Eds.), *Developmental disorders: Diagnostic criteria and clinical assessment* (pp. 127–172). Hillsdale, NJ: Lawrence Erlbaum Associates.

Grodinsky, G. (1990). *Assessing frontal lobe functioning in 6 to 11 year old boys with attention deficit disorder.* Unpublished doctoral dissertation, Boston College, Boston.

Grossmann, H. J. (Ed.). (1983). *Classification in mental retardation.* Washington, DC: American Association on Mental Deficiency.

Guevremont, D. C., & Barkley, R. A. (1992). Attention deficit-hyperactivity disorder in children. In S. R. Hooper, G. W. Hynd, & R. E. Mattison (Eds.), *Child psychopathology: Diagnostic criteria and clinical assessment.* Hillsdale, NJ: Lawrence Erlbaum Associates.

Guilford, J. P. (1967). *The nature of human intelligence.* New York: McGraw-Hill.

Hagan, J. W., & Huntsman, N. (1971). Selective attention in mental retardates. *Developmental Psychology, 5,* 151–160.

Haggerty, R. J. (1986). The changing nature of pediatrics. In N. A. Krasnegor, J. D. Arasteh, & M. F. Cataldo (Eds.), *Child health behavior: A behavioral pediatrics perspective* (pp. 9–16). New York: John Wiley & Sons.

Hall, J. W., III, Baer, J. E., Byrn, A., Wurm, F. C., Henry, M. M., Wilson, D. S., & Prentice, C. H. (1993). Audiologic assessment and management of central auditory processing disorder (CAPD). *Seminars in Hearing, 14,* 254–263.

Harrison, A., Serafica, F., & McAdoo, H. (1984). Ethnic families of color. In R. D. Parke (Ed.), *Review of child development research* (Vol. 7) (pp. 329–371). Chicago: University of Chicago Press.

Hauser, S. L., DeLong, G. R., & Rosman, N. P. (1975). Pneumographic findings in the infantile autism syndrome: A correlation with temporal lobe disease. *Brain, 98,* 667–688.

Haynes, S. (1985). Developmental apraxia of speech: Symptoms and treatment. In D. F. Johns (Ed.), *Clinical Management of Neurogenic Communicative Disorders.* Boston: Little, Brown & Co.

Holborrow, P. L., Berry, P., & Elkins, J. (1984). Prevalence of hyperkinesis: A comparison of three rating scales. *Journal of Learning Disabilities, 17,* 411–417.

Hooper, S. R., & Willis, W. G. (1989). *Learning disability subtyping. Neuropsychological foundations, conceptual models, and issues in clinical differentiation.* New York: Springer-Verlag.

Horn, J. L. (1985). Remodeling old models of intelligence. In B. Wolman (Ed.), *Handbook of intelligence* (pp. 267–300). New York: Wiley.

Howlin, P. (1989). Changing approaches to communication training with autistic children. *British Journal of Disorders of Communication, 24,* 151–168.

Hyman, S. L., Batshaw, M. L., Porter, C. A., Page, T. J., Iwata, B. A., Kissel, R., & O'Brien, S. (1987). Behavioral management of feeding disorders in children with urea cycle and organic acid disorders.

Journal of Pediatrics, *111*(4), 558–562.

Hynd, G. W., & Hooper, S. R. (1992). *Neurological basis of childhood psychopathology*. Newbury Park, CA: Sage Publications.

Ingram, D. (1976). *Phonological disability in children*. New York: Elsevier.

Interagency Committee on Learning Disabilities (1987). *Learning disabilities: A report to the U. S. Congress*. Washington, DC: Author.

Irvin, N. A., Kennell, J. H., & Klaus, M. H. (1982). Caring for parents of the infant with a congenital malformation. In M. H. Klaus & J. H. Kennell (Eds.), *Parent Infant Bonding* (pp. 227–258). St. Louis: Mosby.

Iwata, B. A., Dorsey, M. F., Slifer, K. J., Bauman, K. E., Richman, G. S. (1982). Toward a functional analysis of self-injury. *Analysis and Intervention in Developmental Disabilities*, *2*, 3–20.

Jay, S. M., Elliot, C. H., Ozolins, M., & Olson, R. A. (1982, August). *Behavioral management of children's distress during painful medical procedures*. Paper presented at the American Psychological Association Convention, Washington, DC.

Jelm, J. (1990). *Oral-Motor/Feeding Rating Scale*. Tuscon: Therapy Skill Builders.

Jerger, J. (1992). Can age-related decline in speech understanding be explained by peripheral hearing loss? *Journal of the American Academy of Audiology*, *3*, 33–38.

Jerger, J. F., & Chmiel, R. (1993). Some factors affecting assessment of hearing handicap in the elderly. *Journal of the American Academy of Audiology*, *4*, 249–257.

Jerger, S., Oliver, T. A., & Martin, R. C. (1990). Evaluation of adult aphasics with the Pediatric Speech Intelligibility Test. *Journal of the American Academy of Audiology*, *1*, 89–100.

Joint Committee on Infant Hearing (1991). 1990 position statement. *Asha*, *33* (Suppl. 5), 3–6.

Kanner, L. (1943). Autistic disturbances of affective contact. *Nervous Child*, *2*(1), 217–250.

Kanner, L. (1946). Irrelevant and metaphorical language in early infantile autism. *American Journal of Psychiatry*, *103*, 242–246.

Kantor, D. (1983). The structural-analytic approach to the treatment of family developmental crisis. In J. Hansen & H. Liddle (Eds.), *Clinical implications of the family life cycle* (pp. 12–34). Rockville, MD: Aspen.

Kaufman, A. S. (1979). *Intelligent testing with the WISC-R*. New York: John Wiley and Sons.

Kedesdy, J. H., & Russo, D. C. (1988). Behavioral medicine with the developmentally disabled: Major issues and challenges. In D.C. Russo

& J.H. Kedesdy (Eds.), *Behavioral medicine with the developmentally disabled* (pp. 1–18). New York: Plenum Press.

Kemp, D. T., & Ryan, S. (1993). The use of transient evoked otoacoustic emissions in neonatal hearing screening. *Seminars in Hearing, 14,* 30–44.

Kenny, D., Koheil, R., Greenberg, J., Reid, D., Milner, M., Moran, R., & Judd, P. (1989). Development of a multidisciplinary feeding profile for children who are dependent feeders. *Dysphagia, 4,* 16–28.

Kent, R. D. (1976). Anatomical and neuromuscular maturation of the speech mechanism: evidence from acoustic studies. *Journal of Speech and Hearing Research, 19,* 421.

Kirby, J. R., & Das, J. P. (1977). Reading achievement, IQ, and simultaneous-successive processing. *Journal of Educational Psychology, 69,* 564–570.

Kirk, S. A. (1963). Behavioral diagnosis and remediation of learning disabilities. In *Proceeding of the Conference on* Exploration into the Problems of the Perceptually *Handicapped Child.* Chicago: Perceptually Handicapped Children.

Klanderman, J. W., & Kaplan, R. J. (1982, October). *Sequential-simultaneous processing of trainable mentally handicapped children and adolescents.* Paper presented at the meeting of the National Academy of Neuropsychologists, Atlanta, GA.

Knox, S. (1974). A play scale. In M. Reilly (Ed.), *Play as exploratory learning* (pp. 247–266). Beverly Hills: Sage Publications.

Koegel, R. L., Dunlap, G., Richman, G. S., & Dyer, K. (1981). The use of specific orienting cues for teaching discrimination tasks. *Analysis and Intervention in Developmental Disabilities, 1,* 187–198.

Koegel, R. L., Koegel, L. K., & Surratt, A. (1992). Language intervention and disruptive behavior in preschool children with autism. *Journal of Autism and Developmental Disorders, 22*(2), 141–153.

Koegel, R. L., O'Dell, M. C., & Koegel, L. K. (1987). A natural language teaching paradigm for nonverbal autistic children. *Journal of Autism and Developmental Disorders, 17,* 187–200.

Koegel, R. L., & Schreibman, L. (1976). Identification of consistent responding to auditory stimuli by a functionally "deaf" autistic child. *Journal of Autism and Childhood Schizophrenia, 6,* 147–156.

Koegel, R. L., & Schreibman, L. (1977). Teaching autistic children to respond to simultaneous multiple cues. *Journal of Experimental Child Psychiatry, 24,* 299–311.

Kolko, D. J., Anderson, L., & Campbell, M. (1980). Sensory preference and overselective responding in autistic children. *Journal of Autism and Developmental Disorders, 10*(3), 259–271.

Krantz, P. J., & McClannahan, L. E. (1993). Teaching children with autism to initiate to peers: Effects of a script-fading procedure. *Journal of Applied Behavior Analysis, 26*(1), 121–132.

Krasnegor, N. A., Arasteh, J. D., & Cataldo, M. F. (Eds.). (1986). *Child health behavior: A behavioral pediatrics perspective*. New York: John Wiley & Sons, Inc.

Lally, M., & Nettelbeck, T. (1977). Intelligence, reaction time, and inspection time. *American Journal of Mental Deficiency, 82*, 79–83.

Lambie, R., & Daniels-Mohring, D. (1993). *Family systems within educational contexts: Understanding students with special needs*. Denver: Love Publishing Company.

Larsen, S., & Hammill, D. (1989). *Test of Legible Handwriting*. Austin, TX: PRO-ED.

Leonard, L. B. (1989). Language learnability and specific language impairment in children. *Applied Psycholinguistics, 2*, 89–118.

Logemann, J. (1983). *Evaluation and treatment of swallowing disorders*. San Diego: College-Hill Press.

Long, C. II, Conrad, P. W., Hall, E. A., & Furler, S. L. (1970). Intrinsic-extrinsic muscle control of the hand in power and precision handling. *Journal of Bone and Joint Surgery, 52*-A, 853–867.

Lou, H. C., Hendricksen, L., & Bruhn, P. (1984). Focal cerebral hypoperfusion in children with dysphasia and/or attention deficit disorder. *Archives of Neurology, 41*, 825–829.

Lou, H. C., Hendriksen, L., Bruhn, P., Borner, H., & Nielsen, J. (1989). Striatal dysfunction in attention deficit disorder and hyperkinetic disorder. *Archives of Neurology, 46*, 48–52.

Lovaas, O. I., Schreibman, L., Koegel, R. L., & Rehm, R. (1971). Selective responding by autistic children to multiple sensory input. *Journal of Abnormal Psychology, 77*, 211–222.

Luria, A. R. (1966). *Human brain and psychological process* (B. Haigh, Trans.). New York: Harper & Row.

Luria, A. R. (1970). Functional organization of the brain. *Scientific American, 222*, 66–78.

Lyon, G. R., & Watson, B. (1981). Empirically derived subgroups of learning disabled readers: Diagnostic characteristics. *Journal of Learning Disabilities, 14*, 256–261.

Mace, F. C., Page, T. J., Ivancic, M. T., & O'Brien, S. (1986). Analysis of environmental determinants of aggression and disruption in mentally retarded children. *Applied Research in Mental Retardation, 7*, 203–221.

Magrun, W. M. (1989). *Evaluating Movement & Posture Disorganization in Dyspraxic Children: A Criteria-based Reference Format for Observing and Analyzing Motor Incoordination in Learning Disabled Children*. N. Syracuse, NY: Advanced Therapeutics.

Mariani, M. A. (1990). *The nature of neuropsychological functioning in preschool-age children with attention-deficit hyperactivity disorder.* Unpublished doctoral dissertation, Boston College.

Marshall, P. (1989). Attention deficit disorder and allergy: A neurochemical model of the relation between the illnesses. *Psychological Bulletin, 106,* 434–446.

Mattis, S., French, J. H., & Rapin, I. (1975). Dyslexia in children and young adults: Three independent neuropsychological syndromes. *Developmental Medicine and Child Neurology, 17,* 150–163.

Maxon, A. B., & Brackett, D. (1992). *The hearing-impaired child: Infancy through high school years.* Boston: Andover Medical Publishers.

Maxon, A. B., & Smaldino, J. (1991). Hearing aid management for children. *Seminars in Hearing, 12,* 365–378.

McLaren, J., & Bryson, S. E. (1987). Review of recent epidemiological studies of mental retardation: Prevalence, associated disorders, and etiology. *American Journal of Mental Retardation, 92*(3), 243–254.

Merril, E. C. (1992). Attentional, resource demands of stimulus encoding for persons with and without mental retardation. *American Journal of Mental Retardation, 97,* 87–98.

Minihan, P. M., & Dean, D. H. (1990). Meeting the needs for health services of persons with mental retardation living in the community. *American Journal of Public Health, 80*(9), 1043–1048.

Minshew, N. J., & Payton, J. B. (1988). New perspectives in autism, Part 1: The clinical spectrum of autism. *Current Problems in Pediatrics, 18*(11), 566–617.

Minuchin, S. (1974). *Families and family therapy.* Cambridge:Harvard University Press.

Morgan, W. P. (1896). A case of congenital word-blindness. *British Medical Journal, 2,* 1978.

Morris, S. (1982). *Pre-Speech Assessment Scale.* Clifton, NJ: J. A. Preston.

Morris, S., & Klein, M. (1987). *Pre-feeding skills: A comprehensive resource for feeding development.* Tuscon: Therapy Skill Builders.

Mutti, M., Sterling, H., & Spalding, N. (1978). *Quick Neurological Screening Test* (rev. ed.). Los Angeles: Western Psychological Services.

Naidoo, S. (1972). *Specific dyslexia.* New York: Wiley.

National Institutes of Health, U.S. Department of Health and Human Services, Public Health Service. (1991). *Treatment of destructive behaviors in persons with developmental disabilities.* National Institutes of Health Consensus Development Conference. Bethesda, MD: NIH.

Nazzaro, J. N. (Ed.). (1981). *Culturally diverse exceptional children in school*. Washington, DC: National Institute of Education.

Nebes, R. D. (1975). Hemispheric specilization in commissurotomized man. *Pyschological Bulletin, 81*, 1–14.

Neef, N. A., Parrish, J. M., Hannigan, K. F., Page, T. J., & Iwata, B. A. (1989). Teaching self-catheterization skills to children with neurogenic bladder complications. *Journal of Applied Behavior Analysis, 22*(3), 237–243.

Nehring, A., Nehring, E., Bruni, J., & Randolph, P. (1992). *Learning Accomplishment Profile-Diagnostic Standardized Assessment* (LAP-D) (rev. ed.). Lewisville, NC: Kaplan Press.

Nelson, H. E., & Warrington, E. K. (1974). Developmental spelling retardation and its relation to other cognitive abilities. *British Journal of Psychology, 65*, 265–274.

Nettlebeck, T., & Brewer, N. (1981). Studies of mild mental retardation and timed performance. In N. R. Ellis (Ed.), *International review of research in mental retardation* (Vol. 10) (pp. 62–106). New York: Academic Press.

Nippold, M. (1988). Figurative language. In M. A. Nippold (Ed.), *Later language development* (pp. 49–96). Boston: Little, Brown and Company.

Norton, S. J. (1993). Application of transient evoked otoacoustic emissions to pediatric populations. *Ear and Hearing, 14*, 64–73.

Nozza, R. J., Bluestone, C. D., Kardatzke, D., & Bachman, R. (1992). Towards the validation of aural acoustic immittance measures for diagnosis of middle ear effusion in children. *Ear and Hearing, 13*, 442–453.

Ogle, J. W. (1867). *Aphasia, apraxia, aphasia: Their value in cerebral localization* (2nd ed.). New York: Hoeber.

Oller, D. K. (1980). The emergence of speech sounds in infancy. In G. H. Yeni-Komshian, J. F. Kavanagh, & C. A. Ferguson (Eds.), *Child phonology* (Vol. 1) (pp. 93–112). New York: Academic Press.

Omenn, G. S. (1973). Genetic issues in the syndrome of minimal brain dysfunction. *Seminars in Psychiatry, 5*, 5–17.

Page, T., Iwata, B., & Neef, N. (1976). Teaching pedestrian skills to retarded persons: Generalization from the classroom to the natural environment. *Journal of Applied Behavior Analysis, 9*(4), 433–444.

Palmer, S., & Horn, S. (1978). Feeding problems in children. In S. Palmer & S. Ekvall (Eds.), *Pediatric nutrition in developmental disorders* (pp. 107–129). Springfield, IL: Charles C. Thomas.

Parker, L. H., Cataldo, M. F., Bourland, G., Emurian, C. S., Corbin, R. J., & Page, J. M. (1984). Operant treatment of orofacial dysfunction in neuromuscular disorders. *Journal of Applied Behavior Analysis*,

17(4), 413–427.

Parrish, J. M., Hannigan, K. F., Page, T. J, & Iwata, B. A. (1989). Teaching self-catheterization skills to children with neurogenic bladder complications. *Journal of Applied Behavior Analysis, 22*(3), 237–243.

Paul, R., & Alforde, S. (1993). Grammatical morpheme acquisition in 4-year-olds with normal, impaired, and late-developing language. *Journal of Speech and Hearing Research, 36,* 1271–1275.

Pavio, A. (1976). Concerning dual-coding and simultaneous-successive processing. *Canadian Psychological Review, 17,* 69–71.

Pelco, L. E., Kissel, R. C., Parrish, J. M., & Miltenberger, R. G. (1987). Behavioral management of oral medication administration difficulties among children: A review of the literature with case illustrations. *Journal of Developmental and Behavioral Pediatrics, 8*(2), 90–96.

Pelham, W. S. (1982). Childhood hyperactivity: Diagnosis, etiology, nature and treatment. In R. Gatchel, A. Baum, & J. Singer (Eds.), *Handbook of psychology and health.* Volume 1: *Clinical psychology and behavioral medicine: Overlapping disciplines* (pp. 261–327). New York: Lawrence Erlbaum.

Pennington, B. F. (1991). *Diagnosing learning disorders: A neuropsychological framework.* New York: Guilford.

Phelps, J., Stempel, L., & Speck, G. (1984). *The Children's Handwriting Evaluation Scale.* Dallas: CHES (6031 St. Andrews, 75205).

Phelps, J., & Stempel, L. (1987). *The Children's Handwriting Evaluation Scale for Manuscript Writing.* Dallas: CHES (6031 St. Andrews, 75205).

Picton, T. W. (1991). Clinical usefulness of auditory evoked potentials: A critical evaluation. *Journal of Speech-Language Pathology and Audiology/Revue d'othophonie et d'audiologie, 15,* 3–29.

Pirozzolo, F. J. (1979). *The neuropsychology of developmental reading disorders.* New York: Praeger Press.

Prizant, B., & Duchan, J. (1981). The functions of immediate echolalia in autistic children. *Journal of Speech and Hearing Research, 46,* 241–250.

Public Law 94–142. (1975). Education for All Handicapped Children Act. Washington, DC: U.S. Government Printing Office.

Public Law 99–457. (1986). Education of the Handicapped Act Amendments of 1986. Washington, DC: U.S. Government Printing Office.

Ricks, D. M., & Wing, L. (1975). Language, communication, and the use of symbols in normal and autistic children. *Journal of Autism and Childhood Schizophrenia, 5*(3), 191–221.

Rincover, A. (1978). Variables affecting stimulus fading and discriminative responding in psychotic children. *Journal of Abnormal Psychology, 87,* 541–553.

Rincover, A., & Ducharme, J. M. (1987). Variables influencing stimulus overselectivity and "tunnel vision" in developmentally delayed children. *American Journal of Mental Deficiency, 91,* 422–430.

Rincover, A., & Koegel, R. L. (1975). Setting generality and stimulus control in autistic children. *Journal of Applied Behavior Analysis, 8*(3), 235–246.

Roeltgen, D. (1985). Agraphia. In K. M. Heilman, & E. Valenstein (Eds.), *Clinical neuropsychology* (2nd ed.) (pp. 75–96). New York: Oxford University Press.

Rosenbloom, L., & Horton, M. E. (1971). The maturation of fine prehension in young children. *Developmental Medicine and Child Neurology, 13,* 3–8.

Ross, D. M., & Ross, S. A. (1982). *Hyperactivity: Current issues, research and theory* (2nd ed.). New York: Wiley.

Roth, F., & Spekman, N. (1986). Narrative discourse: Spontaneously generated stories of learning-disabled and normal achieving students. *Journal of Speech and Hearing Disorders, 51,* 8–23.

Rourke, B. P. (1989). *Nonverbal learning disabilities: The syndrome and the model.* New York: Guilford Press.

Rourke, B. P., & Finlayson, M. A. J. (1978). Neuropsychological significance of variations in patterns of academic performance: Verbal and visual-spatial abilities. *Journal of Abnormal Child Psychology, 6,* 121–133.

Rourke, B. P., & Strang, J. D. (1978). Neuropsychological significance of variations in patterns of academic performance: Motor, psychomotor, and tactile-perceptual abilities. *Journal of Pediatric Psychology, 3,* 62–66.

Rumsey, J. M. (1985). Conceptual problem-solving in highly verbal, nonretarded autistic men. *Journal of Autism and Developmental Disorders, 15*(1), 23–36.

Russo, D. C., & Kedesdy, J. H. (1988). *Behavioral medicine with the developmentally disabled.* New York: Plenum Press.

Rutter, M. (1965). The influence of organic and emotional factors on the origins, nature and outcome of childhood psychosis. *Developmental Medicine and Child Neurology, 7,* 518–528.

Rutter, M., & Lockyer, L. (1967). A five to fifteen year follow-up study of infantile psychosis: I. Description of sample. *British Journal of Psychiatry, 113,* 1169–1182.

Rutter, M., & Schopler, E. (1987). Autism and pervasive developmental disorders: Concepts and diagnostic issues. *Journal of Autism and Developmental Disorders, 17*(2), 159–186.

Sandler, A. D., Watson, T. E., Footo, M., Levine, M. D., Coleman, W. L., & Hooper, S. R. (1992). Neurodevelopmental study of writing disorders in middle childhood. *Developmental and Behavioral Pediatrics, 13*, 17–23.

Satz, P., & Morris, R. (1981). Learning disabilities subtypes: A review. In F. J. Pirozzolo, & M. C. Wittrock (Eds.), *Neuropsychological and cognitive processes in reading* (pp. 109–141). New York: Academic Press.

Schafer, D., & Moersch, M. (Eds.). (1981). *Developmental Programming for Infants and Young Children.* Ann Arbor: The University of Michigan Press.

Schneck, C., & Henderson, A. (1990). Descriptive analysis of the developmental progression of grip position for pencil and crayon control in nondysfunctional children. *American Journal of Occupational Therapy, 10*, 893–900.

Schneider, W., & Shiffrin, R. M. (1977). Controlled and automatic human information processing: I. Detection, search, and attention. *Psychological Review, 84*, 1–66.

Schreibman, L., Charlop, M. H., & Koegel, R. L. (1982). Teaching autistic children to use extra-stimulus prompts. *Journal of Experimental Child Psychology, 33*, 475–491.

Schreibman, L., & Lovaas, O. I. (1973). Overselective response to social stimuli by autistic children. *Journal of Abnormal Psychology, 1*(2), 152–168.

Schroeder, S. R., Rojahn, J., Oldenquist, A. (1991). Treatment of destructive behaviors among people with mental retardation and developmental disabilities: Overview of the problem. In National Institutes of Health Consensus Conference Report on *Treatment of destructive behaviors in persons with developmental disabilities* (pp. 125–171). Bethesda, MD: NIH.

Schwartz, G. E., & Weiss, S. M. (1978). Yale Conference on Behavioral Medicine: A proposed definition and statement of goals. *Journal of Behavioral Medicine, 1*, 3–12.

Scott, C. M. (1988). Spoken and written syntax. In M. A. Nippold (Ed.), *Later language development* (pp. 49–96). Boston: Little, Brown and Company.

Seligman, M., & Darling, R. B. (1989). *Ordinary families, special children: A systems approach to childhood disability.* New York: The Guilford Press.

Shea, T. M., & Bauer, A. M. (1991). *Parents and teachers of children with exceptionalities: A handbook for collaboration.* Boston: Allyn & Bacon.

Simpson, R. L. (1990). *Conferencing parents of exceptional children* (2nd ed.). Austin, TX: PRO-ED.

Slifer, K. J., Ivancic, M. T., Parrish, J. M., Page, T. J., & Burgio, L. D.

(1986). Assessment and treatment of multiple behavior problems exhibited by a profoundly retarded adolescent. *Journal of Behavior Therapy and Experimental Psychiatry, 17*(3), 203–213.

Sloman, L. (1991). Use of medication in pervasive developmental disorders. *Psychiatric Clinics of North America, 14*(1), 165–182.

Spearman, C. E. (1927). *The abilities of man.* New York: Macmillan.

Sperber, R., & McCauley, C. (1984). Semantic processing efficiency in the mentally retarded. In P. H. Brooks, R. Sperber, & C. McCauley (Eds.), *Learning and cognition in the mentally retarded* (pp. 141–163). Hillsdale, NJ: Lawrence Erlbaum Associates.

Stach, B. A., & Loiselle, L. H. (1993). Central auditory processing disorder: Diagnosis and management in a young child. *Seminars in Hearing, 14,* 288–295.

Stanovich, K. E. (1978). Information processing in mentally retarded individuals. In N. R. Ellis (Ed.), *International review of research in mental retardation* (Vol. 9) (pp. 29–60). New York: Academic Press.

Stark, R. E. (1980). Stages of speech development in the first year of life. In G. H. Yeni-Komshian, J. F. Kavanagh, and C. A. Ferguson (Eds.), *Child phonology* (Vol. 1). New York: Academic Press.

Sternberg, R. J. (1986). *Intelligence applied: Understanding and increasing your intellectual skills.* San Diego: Harcourt, Brace, Jovanovich, Inc.

Sternberg, R. J. (1988). *The triarchic mind: A New theory of human intelligence.* New York: Penguin Books.

Stilwell, J. (1987). The development of manual midline crossing in 2- to 6-year old children. *American Journal of Occupational Therapy, 41,* 783–789.

Stott, D., Moyes, F., & Henderson, S. (1985). *Diagnosis and remediation of handwriting problems.* Ontario, Canada: Brook Educational Publishing.

Stuber W., Dehne, P., Miedaner, J., & Romero, P. (1987). *Milani-Comparetti Motor Development Screening Test Manual* (rev. ed.) Omaha: Meyer Rehabilitation Institute.

Summers, J. A., Rincover, A., & Feldman, M. A. (1993). Comparison of extra- and within-stimulus prompting to teach prepositional discriminations to preschool children with developmental disabilities. *Journal of Behavioral Education, 3*(3), 287–298.

Sutter, E. G., Bishop, P. C., & Batten, R. R. (1986). Factor similarities between traditional psychoeducational and neuropsychological test batteries. *Journal of Psychoeducational Assessment, 4,* 73–82.

Sweeney, J. E., & Rourke, B. P. (1978). Neuropsychological significance of phonetically accurate and phonetically inaccurate spelling errors of younger and older retarded spellers. *Brain and Language, 6,* 212–225.

Tannock R., Purvis, K. L., & Schachar, R. J. (1993). Narrative abilities in children with attention deficit hyperactivity disorder and normal peers. *Journal of Abnormal Child Psychology, 21,* 103–117.

Thorndike, E. L. (1927). *The measurement of intelligence.* New York: Bureau of Publications, Teachers College, Columbia University.

Thurstone, L. L. (1938). Primary mental abilities. *Psychometric Monographs,* No. 1.

Tomporowski, P. D., Hayden, A. M., & Applegate, B. (1990). Effects of background event rate on sustained attention of mentally retarded and nonretarded adults. *American Journal of Mental Retardation, 94,* 499–508.

Turkington, C. (1993, January). New definition of retardation includes the need for support. *APA Monitor,* pp. 26–27.

Turnbull, A. P., & Turnbull, H. R. (1990). *Families, professionals, and exceptionality: A special partnership* (2nd ed.). Columbus, OH: Merrill Publishing Company.

U. S. Office of Education (1977). Assistance to states for education of handicapped children: Procedures for evaluating specific learning disabilities. *Federal Register, 42*(250), 65082–65085.

Varni, J. W. (1983). *Clinical Behavioral Pediatrics: An interdisciplinary biobehavioral approach* (pp. 3–15). New York: Pergamon Press.

Varni, J. W., Bessman, C. A., Russo, D. C., & Cataldo, M. F. (1980). Behavioral management of chronic pain in children: Case study. *Archives of Physical Medicine and Rehabilitation, 61,* 375–379.

Varni, J. W., Walco, G. A., & Wilcox, K. T. (1990). Cognitive biobehavioral assessment and treatment of pediatric pain. In A. M. Gross & R. S. Drabman (Eds.), *Handbook of Clinical Behavioral Pediatrics* (pp. 83–97). New York: Plenum Press.

Vernon, P. E. (1950). *The structure of human abilities.* New York: Wiley.

Vulpe, S. G. (1977). *Vulpe Assessment Battery* (2nd ed.). Downsview, Ontario: National Institute on Mental Retardation.

Wender, P. (1971). *Minimal brain dysfunction in children.* New York: Wiley.

White, K. R., Vohr, B. R., & Behrens, T. R. (1993). Universal newborn hearing screening using transient evoked otoacoustic emissions: Result of the Rhode Island hearing assessment project. *Seminars in Hearing, 14,* 18–29.

Whitehead, W. (1986). Pediatric gastrointestinal disorders. In N. Krasnegor, J. Arasteh & M. Cataldo (Eds.). *Child Health Behavior: A behavioral pediatrics perspective* (pp. 371–393). New York: Wiley & Sons.

Whitehead, W. E., Parker, L. H., Masek, B. J., Cataldo, M. F., & Freeman, J. M. (1981). Biofeedback treatment of fecal incontinence in patients with myelomeningocele. *Developmental Medicine and Child Neurology, 23,* 313–322.

Widen, J. E. (1993). Adding objectivity to infant behavioral audiometry. *Ear and Hearing, 14,* 49–57.

Wilhelm, H., & Lovaas, O. I. (1976). Stimulus overselectivity: A common feature in autism and mental retardation. *American Journal of Mental Deficiency, 81*(1), 26–31.

Wing, L. (1981). Language, social and cognitive impairments in autism and severe mental retardation. *Journal of Autism and Developmental Disorders, 11*(1), 31–44.

Wing, L., & Attwood, A. (1987). Syndromes of autism and atypical development. In D. J. Cohen, & A. M. Donnellan (Eds.), *Handbook of autism and pervasive developmental disorders* (pp. 3–19). New York: Wiley.

Wolf, L., & Glass, R. (1992). Clinical feeding evaluation of infants. In L. Wolf & R. Glass (Eds.), *Feeding and swallowing disorders in infancy: Assessment and management* (pp. 54–57). Tucson: Therapy Skill Builders.

Wolff, P.H. (1968). The serial organization of sucking in the young infant. *Pediatrics, 42,* 943–955.

Wynne, M. K. (1992, October). *Central auditory processing disorders: Paradigms approaching chaos.* Paper presented at the annual convention of the Kansas Speech and Hearing Association, Overland Park, KS.

Zametkin, A. J., & Rapoport, J. L. (1986). Neurobiology of attention deficit disorder with hyperactivity: Where have we come in 50 years? *Journal of the American Academy of Child and Adolescent Psychiatry, 26,* 676–686.

Zeaman, D., & House, B. A. (1979). A review of attention theory. In N. R. Ellis (Ed.), *Handbook of mental deficiency: Psychological theory and research* (2nd ed.) (pp. 63–120). Hillsdale, NJ: Lawrence Erlbaum Associates.

INDEX

A

Afro-American subculture, 156
American Association of Mental
    Retardation, 68–69
Apraxia, 105
Apraxia of speech, prosody, 106
Articulation disorders, 104–105
Articulatory system, 103–105
Assessment
    motor, 54–56. *See also* Examination,
        neurodevelopmental
    oral motor, 55–56
Assessment tools, pediatric, 33
Ataxia, 52–53
Athetosis, 53
Attention-deficit hyperactivity disorder
    (ADHD), 75, 79–81,
    183–186
    definition, 79–80
    etiological theories, 80–81
    impaired language, 114–115
    incidence, 80
    primary disabling conditions, 24
    short-term memory, 18
Audiograms, 90, 92–93

Audiology, 87, 89
    pediatric, 91, 100
Aural (re)habilitation, 100–101
Autism
    behavioral characteristics, 143–144
    behavior problems, 141–146
    behaviors and communication, 144
    and communication disorders, 74
    communication training, 144–146
    echolalia, 116, 143
    impaired language, 115–117
    incidence, 74
    infantile, 23
    language assessment, 87
    overselective responding, 142–143
    prosody, 106
    social-communicative interaction
        training, 145–146

B

Behavioral psychology overview,
    121–124
Behavior problems, 121–151
    analytic approach application,
        127–133

Behavior problems *(continued)*
  antecedent-behavior-consequence
    approach application, 127–133
  autism, 141–146
  behavior analysis, 124–127
  behavior relationship (response
    classes), 137–140
  differential reinforcement of 0 rate
    (DRO), 133
  functional analysis, 125, 133–137
  graphic display, 126–129
  incidence nationally, 123

C

Central nervous system damage,
    primary disabling conditions,
    25–26
Cerebral palsy
  hypertonus, 49
  hypotonic and/or ataxic, 53
  incidence, ix
  neurological involvement extent, 28
  primary disabling conditions, 22
  and respiratory system, 102
Chorea, 54
Cleft palate, 103
  articulation disorders, 105
Cognition
  bodily-kinesthetic intelligence, 64
  componential elements, 65–67
  contextual elements, 65–67
  and emotional disturbance, 67–68
  and environment, 68
  experiential elements, 65–67
  Gardner's model, 63–65
  Guilford's Structure of Intellect
    (SOI) model, 60–61
  intrapersonal/interpersonal intelli-
    gence, 64
  IQ measure usefulness, 60
  linguistic intelligence, 63
  logical-mathematical intelligence, 63
  Luria's neuropsychological model,
    61–63
  musical intelligence, 63–64
  and sensory impairment, 67

Cognition *(continued)*
  simultaneous information processing,
    62
  spatial intelligence, 64
  Sternberg's triarchic model, 65–67
  Structure of Intellect (SOI),
    Guilford's model, 60–61
  successive information processing, 62
  triarchic theory, 65–67
Cognitive impairment, 59–83
Cognitively based disorders, 68–81
  assessment strategies, 81–82
  attention-deficit hyperactivity
    disorder (ADHD), 79–81
  autism, 73–74
  clinical issues, 82
  communication disorders, 72–74
  developmental levels, 82
  learning disorder, 74–79
  mental retardation, 68–72
  reliable assessment, 82
Communication disorders
  autistic disorder, 73–74
  behavioral indicators, 73
  primary disabling conditions, 22–23
Cultural differences, 155–156

D

Development
  cup drinking, 45
  fine motor milestones, 10
  Gesell developmental domains, 2–3, 68
  grammatical, 107–109
  grasp muscle control, 39–40
  gross motor milestones, 8
  language, 107–119
    expressive/receptive milestones, 9
  manipulation muscle control, 41–42
  motor function, normal
    fine function, 35–42
    gross function, 30–35
    oral motor function, 42–45
  munching/chewing muscle control,
    44–45
  posture transition muscle control, 35
  pragmatic (social) language, 111–113

Development *(continued)*
  prone muscle control, 30
  reach muscle control, 38
  release muscle control, 40
  semantic, 109–111
  sitting muscle control, 34
  spoon feeding, 45
  standing muscle control, 34–35
  sucking muscle control, 42
  supine muscle control, 34
  swallowing, 42–43
  visual perceptual milestones, 10
  walking muscle control, 35
Diagnosis, and physician as generalist, 2–3
Dyscoordination, 52–53
Dyslexia, language assessment, 87

E

Echolalia, 16, 116, 143
Education of the Handicapped Act (EHA), 57
Encephalopathy, 3
Examination, neurodevelopmental, 10–19, 172–173, 181–184. *See also* Assessment, motor
  associated deficits, 26–27
  attention-deficit hyperactivity disorder (ADHD), 18
  fine motor function, 17
  Gesell drawings, 14–15
  gross motor function, 16–17
  interpretation factors, 20–21
  language functioning, 15–16
    comprehension, 15–16
    echolalia, 16
    receptive/expressive, 16
  mirror movements, 18
  oral motor function, 17
  patterns of primary conditions, 25–26
  Peabody Picture Vocabulary Test-Revised (PPVT-R), 15–16
  primary disabling conditions, 22–24
  problem solving, 12–15
  psychosocial deprivation, 20–21
  rapport building, 11

Examination *(continued)*
  and screening instruments, 10–11
  short-term memory, 18
  soft neurological signs, 17–18
  synkinesias, 18
  unrecognized sensory deficits, 20–21
  visual perceptual, 12–15

F

Family
  affection needs, 161
  concomitant effects, 155
  cultural differences, 155–156
  daily care needs, 159
  developmental patterns, 20
  education/vocational needs, 161
  and exceptionality characteristics, 154–155
  explaining diagnosis to parents, 166–168
  family life cycle, 161–163
  fine motor questionnaire, 36–38
  gross motor questionnaire, 32
  and hearing impairment, 100–101
  and history, 6–10, 16
  interaction within, 156–158
  medical costs, 159
  oral motor questionnaire, 43–44
  parental reaction to disability diagnosis
    adaptation/adjustment, 165
    ambivalence, 164
    anger, 165
    denial, 164
    guilt, 164–165
    rejection of situation, 165–166
    shopping behavior, 165–166
    sorrow, chronic, 165
  parental subsystem, 157–158
  recreation needs, 160
  self-identity needs, 160
  sibling subsystem, 158
  socialization needs, 160
  spousal subsystem, 157
Fine motor skills, 10

Fluency (stuttering), 106–107
  referral indicators, 106

G

Grammatical development, 107–109
Gross motor skill, 8

H

Hearing impairment, 87–101
  American Sign Language, 91
  assessment
    brain stem-evoked response
      (BSER) audiometry, 99
    infant/child preferred physiological
      measures, 99–100
    otoacoustic emission (OAE)
      testing, 99–100
    physiological measures, 99–100
    tympanometry (immittance
      measure), 98–99
  audibility, speech, 90
  audiograms, 90, 92–93
  auditory training, 100
  aural (re)habilitation, 100–101
  central auditory processing disorders,
    94
  conductive, 92
    loss indicators, 88–89
    overview, 91
  educational needs, 96–98
  and family, 100–101
  FM systems, 100
  hearing aids, 91
  mixed loss, 94, 95
  prosody, 106
  screening, universal, 87–88
  sensorineural, 90, 93, 100
    loss indicators, 88–89
    overview, 91
  severity and effect, 96–98
  sign language, 100–101
  speech-language remediation, 100
History
  neurodevelopmental, 3–10, 171–172,
    177–181

History (continued)
  parents as historians, 6–7, 16
History, neurodevelopmental, 7–10.
    See also Development
  age-equivalent descriptors, 7, 8
  as deficit compendium, 7
Hypertonus
  cerebral palsy, 49
  deficiencies, 46–47
  oral motor abnormalities, 48
  posture, 47–48
  reach, grasp, release, 48
Hypotonus
  deficiencies, 48–50
  oral motor abnormalities, 51–52
  posture, 50–51

I

Impaired language development,
    113–119
  attention-deficit hyperactivity
    disorder (ADHD), 114–115
  autism, 115–117
  learning disability, 118–119
  mental retardation, 114
  specific language impairment (SLI),
    117–118
Individualized education plan (IEP),
    154
Individualized education program
    (IEP), 57
Individualized family service plan
    (IFSP), 57, 153–154
Individuals with Disabilities Act
    (IDEA), 154. See also Public
    Law 101-476 (PL 101-476)
Interdisciplinary, and physician as
    generalist, 2–3
Intervention, 56–57

L

Labor/delivery risk factors, 5
Language impairment
  identification, 86–87
  terminology, 86

Language overview, 107–119. See also
    Impaired language development
    grammatical development, 107–109
    pragmatic development, 111–113
    semantic development, 109–111
Language skills, 9
Laryngeal system, 102
Laryngoscopy, 102
Learning disability
    impaired language, 118–119
    incidence, ix
    mirror movement, 18
    primary disabling conditions, 23–24
    synkinesias, 18
Learning disorder, 74–79
    arithmetic subtypes, 78–79
    reading subtypes, 76
    spelling subtypes, 76–77
    written language subtypes, 77–78

M

Medical care, behavioral procedures
    increasing compliance, 149
Memory, 69–72
    auditory assessment, 19
    short term
        assessment, 18–19
        and attention-deficit hyperactivity
            disorder (ADHD), 18
Mental retardation, 68–72
    attentional deficits, 70–71
    cognitive models, 69–72
    definition, 68–69
    identification issues, 68–69
    impaired language, 114
    incidence, ix
    medical care and behavioral
        psychology, 148
    and memory, 69–72
    neurological involvement extent, 27
    primary disabling conditions, 22
    prosody, 106
    rehearsal strategy efficiency, 71
    sensory and perceptual processing,
        short-term, 70
    skill retention, 72

Mexican-American subculture, 156
Milestones
    fine motor, 10, 31
    gross motor, 8, 31
    language, expressive/receptive, 9
    oral motor, 31
    visual perceptual, 10
Minimal brain dysfunction (MBD),
        primary disabling conditions, 24
Motor dysfunction
    hypertonus, 46–48
    hypotonus, 48–51
    mixed tonal abnormalities, 51–52
    patterns, dyscoordination/extraneous
        movements, 52–54
    tonal difficulties, 46–52
Motor function, normal, gross
        function, 30–42
Motor imparment, damage areas, 29–30

N

Neonatal risk factors, 5
Neurodevelopmental history. See
        History, neurodevelopmental
Neurodevelopmental history taking,
        7–10

O

Occupational therapy, 56–57

P

Parents. See Family
*Peabody Picture Vocabulary Test-
        Revised (PPVT-R),* 15–16, 110,
        118
Pervasive developmental disorders
        (PDD), 141–142
Physical therapy, 56–57
Physician
    as generalist, 2–3
    and neurodevelopmental history, 3–4
Pragmatic development, 111–113
Pregnancy risk factors, 5
Prematurity, 20

Prosody, 105–106
Public Law 94-142 (PL 94-142), 57
Public Law 99-457 (PL 99-457), 57,
    153
Public Law 101-476 (PL 101-476),
    154. *See also* Individuals with
    Disabilities Act (IDEA)

R

Resonance system, 102–103
Respiratory system, 101–102
Risk factors, prenatal/perinatal, 4–6

S

Self-management skill teaching,
    149–150
Semantic development, 109–111
Social-adaptive skills, 7
Specific language impairment (SLI),
    117–118
Speech-language pathology, 85, 87,
    89, 104
Speech system overview, 101–107
    articulatory system, 103–105
    fluency (stuttering), 106–107

Speech system overview *(continued)*
    hypernasality, 103
    hyponasality, 103
    laryngeal system, 102
    prosody, 105–106
    resonance system, 102–103
    respiratory system, 101–102
Sternberg Triarchic Abilities Test,
    66–67
Stuttering. *See* Fluency (stuttering)

T

Tools, pediatric assessment, 33

V

Visual perceptual skills, 10

W

*Wechsler Intelligence Scales for
    Children,* 61
*Wechsler Intelligence Scales for
    Children-III,* 67
*Wechsler Preschool and Primary
    Scales of Intelligence,* 61

TOURO COLLEGE LIBRARY